HEALON

HEALON
(SODIUM HYALURONATE)
A GUIDE TO ITS USE
IN OPHTHALMIC SURGERY

Edited by

David Miller, M.D.
Associate Professor of Ophthalmology
Harvard Medical School
Ophthalmologist-in-Chief
Beth Israel Hospital
Boston, Massachusetts

Robert Stegmann, M.D.
Professor of Ophthalmology
Medical University of Southern Africa
Chief of Ophthalmology
Garankua Hospital
Pretoria, South Africa

A WILEY MEDICAL PUBLICATION
JOHN WILEY & SONS
New York • Chichester • Brisbane • Toronto • Singapore

Cover photograph: Åke Dyfverman

Library of Congress Cataloging in Publication Data

Main entry under title:

Healon (sodium hyaluronate): a guide to its use in ophthalmic surgery.

    (A Wiley medical publication)
    Includes index.
    1. Hyaluronic acid—Therapeutic use. 2. Vitreous body—Surgery. I. Miller, David, 1931–
II. Stegmann, Robert. III. Series.

RE992.H88H43   1983   617.7'4059   82-13381
ISBN 0-471-09561-3

Printed in the United States of America

10 9 8 7 6 5 4 3 2 1

Contributors

Endre A. Balazs, M.D.
Malcolm P. Aldrich Professor of Ophthalmology
Director, Research Division
Department of Ophthalmology
College of Physicians and Surgeons
Columbia University
New York, New York

Henry M. Clayman, M.D.
Clinical Associate Professor
Department of Ophthalmology
Bascom Palmer Eye Institute
University of Miami School of Medicine
Clinical Professor of Health Sciences
Miami-Dade Community College
Miami, Florida

Ake Holmberg, M.D., D.Sc.
Department of Ophthalmology
Karolinska Hospital
Stockholm, Sweden

Mark S. Jaffe, M.D.
Clinical Instructor
Department of Ophthalmology
Bascom Palmer Eye Institute
University of Miami School of Medicine
Miami, Florida

Norman S. Jaffe, M.D.
Clinical Professor
Department of Ophthalmology
Bascom Palmer Eye Institute
University of Miami School of Medicine
Miami, Florida
Chairman, Department of Ophthalmology
St. Francis Hospital
Miami Beach, Florida

Barry Kusman, M.D.
Attending Ophthalmic Surgeon
St. Joseph's Hospital
El Dorado Hospital
Tucson, Arizona

G. William Lazenby, M.D.
Attending Ophthalmologist
Tarpon Springs General Hospital
Tarpon Springs, Florida

David Miller, M.D.
Associate Professor
Department of Ophthalmology
Harvard Medical School
Ophthalmologist-in-Chief
Beth Israel Hospital
Boston, Massachusetts

Bo Philipsson, M.D., D.Sc.
Department of Ophthalmology
Karolinska Hospital
Stockholm, Sweden

Robert Stegmann, M.D.
Professor
Department of Ophthalmology
Medical University of Southern Africa
Chief of Ophthalmology
Garankua Hospital
Pretoria, South Africa

Staffan Stenkula, M.D.
Department of Ophthalmology
Region Hospital
Örebro, Sweden

Ragnar Törnquist, M.D.
Professor
Department of Ophthalmology
Region Hospital
Örebro, Sweden

Foreword

The story of the development of hyaluronic acid for eye surgery is an exciting example of the power of international cooperation. It was originally identified by a German scientist, and ultimately purified by a Hungarian physician. Its early clinical trials as a vitreous substitute were performed by a Belgian ophthalmologist and later extended by a series of European retinal specialists. Its commercial development was then accomplished by a Swedish pharmaceutical company. In 1977, an American ophthalmologist, in concert with a South African ophthalmologist, demonstrated its clinical usefulness in anterior segment ocular surgery. Their clinical observations on the protective action of hyaluronic acid on the corneal endothelium were confirmed by the morphological studies of a South American ophthalmologist. And so this exciting long-chained polymer, with its astounding viscoelastic and piezoelectric properties, has attracted the enthusiasm and curiosity of scientists and clinicians from all over the world.

Finally, the story of Healon® is the story of scientific courage and determination. It was these qualities that led scientists to pursue their goal for more than two decades in the face of many technical frustrations as well as misunderstandings. It was these same qualities that led clinicians to continue their work in the face of initial skepticism from some of their colleagues.

Now that Healon® has passed most of the tribal rites of acceptance, a book is needed that can show the ophthalmic surgeon how to best take advantage of the remarkable properties of sodium hyaluronate in many operations. Drs. Miller and Stegmann have prepared such a book. I am sure readers will benefit from it.

Claes H. Dohlman, M.D.

Professor and Chairman of Ophthalmology
Harvard Medical School
Chief of Ophthalmology
Massachusetts Eye and Ear Infirmary
Boston, Massachusetts

Acknowledgments

The authors would like to extend their special thanks to the following people for their encouragement and help: Dr. L.A.P.A. Munnik, Dr. J. de Beer, Dr. N. Gilliland, Prof. T. Dunston, Dr. Gert Lindblad, Mr. Hans Akerblom, Mr. Gunnar Vicstrom, and Dr. Richard Romasz.

We would also like to thank Ms. Linda M. Poole for her tireless efforts in typing the manuscript and Mr. Klaus Wiederkehr for his technical help.

We want to extend a very special thank you to Mr. Len Koppier for his excellent photography.

Finally, we wish to thank our wives, Ane and Renee, for their never-ending understanding and support.

David Miller
Robert Stegmann

Contents

Introduction: Intraocular Lens Implantation with Healon

David Miller

Robert Stegmann

In his anatomy book for laymen, *The Body in Question,* Dr. Jonathan Miller tries to explain the sudden leap in medical progress within the last 25 years (1). He suggests that understanding how the body survives and protects itself from the viewpoint of bioengineering has been responsible for most of our advances. For example, the application of such suggestive metaphors as "the heart acts like a pump" allowed us to consider logical methods for treating a failing heart sensibly. For us in ophthalmology, the concept of the eye as an optical instrument certainly led to scientific refraction.

This bioengineering hypothesis may also explain one of the latest advances in ophthalmic surgery—the introduction of the viscoelastic polymer, sodium hyaluronate (Healon), into the open eye to facilitate all types of eye surgery. The following story may help to illustrate the point.

In the summer of 1976, one of us (DM) implanted his first intraocular lens. It was an ideal case; an 82-year-old man with a perfect right eye and a mature cataract in the left eye. The implant must have touched a large portion of the corneal endothelium during surgery because the cornea remained edematous for about a month. At about that time, the endothelial camera was being introduced to ophthalmology, and Dr. Herbert Kaufman and his colleagues had used the camera to demonstrate that the implant can pull cells from the back of the cornea if

1

contact between the two takes place (2). Would it not be helpful if a thick, physiologic jelly could be found that would protectively coat the cornea as well as push back the vitreous body and iris in the face of an open incision.

These thoughts brought to mind the research of Professor Endre Balazs on hyaluronic acid. After studying vitreous hyaluronic acid for many years, he had developed a process of purifying it from umbilical cord and rooster combs (3). It had been successfully used as a vitreous replacement in the human eye in the late 1960's, and during that same period Professor Claes Dohlman had used it to maintain a leaking anterior chamber. A telephone call to Professor Balazs confirmed the recollections of the late 1960's and brought the events up to date. When it had been observed that an injection of sodium hyaluronate into the knee joints of horses suffering from traumatic arthritis restored normal function, the product developed an exciting commercial potential, and the process was transferred to a Swedish pharmaceutical company. Professor Balazs agreed to have a number of syringes of sodium hyaluronate shipped to our lab. With these samples we were able to implant lenses in one eye of a large series of rabbits using Healon and compare the Healon-treated eyes to implantations in control eyes using air and balanced salt solution. Postoperatively, the Healon-treated eyes showed clearer corneas and fewer complications (4). Probably because hyaluronic acid, the parent molecule, is found in the same basic molecular configuration throughout the evolutionary scale from microbes to humans, immunologically induced inflammation did not occur.

At this stage it was clear that a proper evaluation of the material in humans was needed, and Dr. Robert Stegmann, of Pretoria, South Africa, was chosen to run the trials. Dr. Stegmann was well suited to evaluate the effects of Healon-treated eyes against a control series of implanted eyes. The socialized system of medicine in his country allowed him to hospitalize his patients for one full postoperative month, permitting him to perform slit lamp measurement and check them on alternate days. The results of the study confirmed the protective effect of Healon on endothelial cells (5). As the material was used more extensively, we also found that it maintained the normal anatomic relationship within the eye during repair of eye trauma, glaucoma surgery, and corneal transplantation.

As our enthusiasm soared, Professor Balazs asked others to confirm our findings. Thus, Dr. Frank Polack and his associates at Gainesville, Florida, produced histologic and clinical evidence that Healon protects the cornea from the trauma of implant and instrument touch (6) and produces better results in corneal transplantation. Dr. Lawrence Pape, at Columbia University, was also able to confirm its usefulness in glaucoma and cataract surgery (7). He also showed that Healon could produce a transient rise in intraocular pressure postoperatively and suggested it be irrigated out at the end of surgery. This work was confirmed by Drs. Norman Jaffe and John Alpar. Drs. Bo Philipsson and Ake Holmberg demonstrated its usefulness in extracapsular cataract extraction. Dr. G. William Lazenby proved the usefulness of Healon in anterior chamber lens implantation and Drs. Staffan Stenkula and Ragnar Törnquist demonstrated its effectiveness in vitrectomy and repairing difficult retinal detachments. As Professor Balazs looked over the many surgical applications of Healon® (Healonid®), he coined the word "viscosurgery" to describe the helpful effects of a viscoelastic fluid during surgical manipulation of the eye.

At this point, one would have to agree with Dr. Jonathan Miller that only after considering endothelial damage due to implant contact from the bioengineering point of view could the solution of a viscoelastic lubricant be envisaged. Of course, luck also plays a role in discovery. It was certainly lucky for all of us that such a physiologic lubricant was available when we decided we needed it.

REFERENCES

1. Miller, J. *The Body in Question.* New York, Random House, 1978.
2. Kaufman, H.E., Katz, J.I. Endothelial damage from intraocular lens insertion. *Invest. Ophthalmol.* 15:996, 1976.
3. Balazs, E.A., Hultsch, E. Replacement of the vitreous with hyaluronic acid, collagen and other polymers, in Irvine, A., O'Malley, C., (eds): *Advances in Vitreous Surgery.* Springfield, Il, Charles C. Thomas, 1976, pp. 609–611.
4. Miller, D., O'Connor, P. Williams, J. Use of Na-hyaluronate during intraocular lens implantation in rabbits. *Ophthalmic Surg.* 11:19, 1980.
5. Miller, D., Stegmann, R. Use of Na-hyaluronate in anterior segment eye surgery. *Am. Intraocular Imp. Soc. J.* 6:13, 1980.
6. Graue, E.L., Polack, F.M., Balazs, E.A. The protective effect of Na-hyaluronate to corneal endothelium. *Exp. Eye Res.* 31:119, 1980.
7. Pape, L.G., Balazs, E.A. The use of Na-hyaluronate (Healon) in human anterior segment surgery. *Ophthalmology* 87:699, 1980.

1

Sodium Hyaluronate and Viscosurgery

Endre A. Balazs

INTRODUCTION

In the field of medicine, ideas are often born prematurely. That is, when they emerge, technology is not available for their realization and medical thinking is not ready for their acceptance. This was the case with the medical use of sodium hyaluronate. The idea for its use to control bone and cartilage healing was born in 1942 (1,2), only six years after the chemical definition of this important component of the joint (3). But the technology was not available to prepare it in a pure form while maintaining its extremely large molecular size. Neither was medicine ready to accept the concept that a component of the extracellular matrix could be used as a controlling factor of its own regenerative processes by applying it in the same tissue compartments where it naturally occurs.

About 15 years later, the need to fill another extracellular space—the vitreous—with a viscous solution during surgery emerged. Human vitreous itself as a heterotransplant was used, but not very successfully because it was not viscous enough. It was again suggested that pure sodium hyaluronate be used as an internal tamponade because it could be prepared in very viscous and elastic solutions, and, as in the joint, a biologic substance was to be used as a surgical aid in the same tissue compartment where it naturally occurred (4). This time the concept was enthusiastically accepted and the developmental work began.

Completely unexpected problems soon emerged. It turned out that the highly purified, sterile, nonpyrogenic substance prepared from human or animal tissues caused unusual nonantigenic-type inflammation

5

when injected in the eye, joint, or abdominal cavity of various species (5,6,7). It took a decade to develop the necessary reproducible and reliable techniques to prepare the so-called noninflammatory fraction of sodium hyaluronate (NIF-NaHA), which could be applied for the intended use (8). As its experimental use in veterinary and human medicine progressed, the concept of viscosurgery was born. What 10 years earlier was only a sketchy idea now became a well-defined medical concept ready for a broad application.

We are only at the beginning of what was called 10 years ago "matrix engineering" (9), the medical manipulation of the extracellular matrix with its own macromolecular components to improve and control the regenerative and even developmental processes of the musculoskeletal and circulatory systems of the body. Many years passed between the first product of matrix engineering—the use of impure collagen (catgut) for surgical sutures—and the second one—the replacement of the vitreous and aqueous humors with sodium hyaluronate. Indeed it will take more time to recognize and use fully the miraculous resources of biologic materials provided by the intercellular matrix of the human and animal body and properly prepare them and use them as tools of matrix engineering.

SODIUM HYALURONATE

In Eye Tissues

Sodium hyaluronate, a large polysaccharide molecule, is present in nearly all connective tissue matrices of vertebrate organisms (10). In some bacteria, it is a capsular polysaccharide. In the human body, it is an important structural element of the skin, subcutaneous and interstitial connective tissues, synovial tissue and fluid, umbilical cord, and the vitreous. Sodium hyaluronate also forms giant molecular complexes with proteoglycans in cartilage. In the eye, sodium hyaluronate was found not only in the vitreous but also in a much lower concentration in the aqueous humor and in the connective tissues of the angle (64).

In the vitreous the concentration of sodium hyaluronate has a considerable variation according to species, age, and topography (11). The highest concentration has been found in the adult cattle and owl monkey vitreous (200–1,000 µg/ml), and the lowest in the adult rabbit, dog, cat, and chicken vitreous (10–60 µg/ml). Between these two extreme values are the adult human and rhesus monkey vitreous (100–400 µg/ml) (12). At birth, the concentration in all species studied is only 1–5% of that of the adult levels. Parallel with the postnatal growth of the eye and the concomitant volume increase of the vitreous, the NaHA concentration slowly increases, reaching maximum levels at sexual maturity. In old age there are only slight variations in the concentration.

Topographically, the NaHA concentration also varies in the vitreous (11). It is always highest in the cortical gel vitreous next to the ciliary body and retina where the cells responsible for its synthesis—the hyalocytes—are located. The concentration is the lowest in the center and anteriorly next to the posterior chamber. The gradient is maintained by the continuous synthesis of NaHA by the hyalocytes and its drainage to the posterior chamber through the annular gap between the lens and the ciliary processes. Since the NaHA molecule is too large to pass through the basal laminae of the retina, ciliary body, and lens, it cannot enter the vitreous from the neighboring tissues nor can it escape except through the basal lamina-free anterior cortical gel to the posterior chamber. From there, diluted by the continuously forming aqueous humor, it is washed into the anterior chamber (Fig. 1).

The NaHA concentration in the anterior chamber of all species investigated is very low (0.5–6.0 µg/ml) (11,13). The only exceptions are owls and fishes, whose anterior chambers are filled with an extremely viscoelastic aqueous humor. This viscoelasticity is dependent on the presence of a relatively high concentration of NaHA in the owl and a NaHA-like molecule (ichthyosan-A) in the fish eye (11). There are some indications that the corneal endothelium in vivo produces NaHA, which then covers it in a very thin layer (75). The function of such a NaHA layer over the corneal endothelium is not understood (64). The NaHA from the anterior chamber passes through the exit passage of the angle through the trabecular meshwork into Schlemm's canal.

Histochemical, physiologic, and, recently, biochemical studies suggest that NaHA and other glycosaminoglycans are present in the connective tissue matrix of the trabeculae and may even be on the surface of the trabecular endothelium (64). It was suggested that NaHA in the angle plays a role in the control of aqueous humor outflow (65) based on the finding that in enucleated eyes of some species, the perfusion of the anterior chamber with NaHA-specific degrading enzymes facilitates the outflow, and that NaHA perfusion decreases it (64,66). In the living eye such an effect was not demonstrated. In fact, one can elevate the NaHA concentration in the anterior chamber of the living rabbit and monkey eye 200 times over the natural level by injecting exogenous large molecular weight NaHA without observing any increase in intraocular pressure (IOP), which would indicate interference with the outflow of aqueous humor. This will be discussed in more detail below.

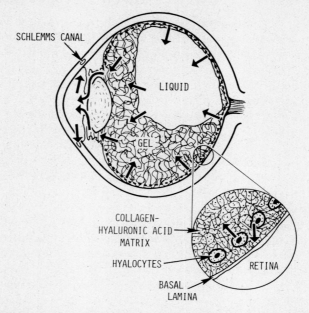

Figure 1. Schematic representation of sodium hyaluronate metabolism in the human vitreous. Arrows indicate the path of the movements of the molecules. In the liquid and gel vitreous the molecules diffuse from the higher to the lower concentration regions. In the posterior chamber, anterior chamber, and the angle the molecules are carried by the flow of aqueous humor. The hyalocytes embedded into the cortical gel excrete the sodium hyaluronate molecules to their extracellular environment: the collagen fibrillar network. (From Balazs and Denlinger: ref. 76).

Viscoelastic Solution

The highly purified sodium hyaluronate is a large polysaccharide molecule with a 2 to 5 million molecular weight. It is a polymer, which means that the long, unbranched chain is made up of 4,700 to 12,000 disaccharide units linked together with a $\beta 1 \to 4$ glucosidic bond. The disaccharide units are sodium glucuronate molecules linked to an *N*-acetylglucosamine molecule by a $\beta 1 \to 3$ glucosidic bond (Fig. 2). According to the best evidence available, this large molecule does not contain other carbohydrates or amino acids, the chain is unbranched, and the chains have no covalent intermolecular bridges. Therefore, in good solvents, the somewhat stiff molecular backbone forms a very flexible, long random coil. Since physiologically balanced salt solution (ionic strength 0.146, pH 7.2) is a fairly good solvent for NaHA, the coil will take up an

Figure 2. The tetrasaccharide segment of a sodium hyaluronate chain. The two monosaccharides *N*-acetyl-D-glucosamine and Na-D-glucuronate are linked together with a β 1 → 4 glucoside bond. The resulting disaccharides are linked together with β 1 → 3 glucoside bonds forming a long unbranched chain.

extremely large volume in the tissues; that is, the overall dimension of the spheroidal domain that the coil occupies in the solvent is in the magnitude of 0.3–0.5 μm. This spongelike molecule contains much water; in other words, its hydrated specific volume is 2–6×10^3 ml/g. This means that, in a solution containing 0.16–0.5 mg NaHA per 1 ml solvent, all the solvent space is occupied. The individual spheroidal domains touch each other, leaving practically no solvent space for other molecules. Therefore, small molecules that can penetrate the spongelike domain of the NaHA will be distributed inside this molecule while those that are too large to penetrate it, such as fibrinogen, collagen, and proteoglycans, will be excluded. (Fig. 3*a*). In both conditions, these molecules will be crowded inside or outside the NaHA molecular domain; therefore, their real concentration and chemical activity will be different from that when they are present in a NaHA-free solution. This phenomenon is called steric exclusion, and its importance in the transport, osmotic activity, and interactions of molecules in the intercellular matrix is well established (10).

As the concentration of these large NaHA molecules is further increased (>0.5 mg/ml), the individual spheroidal molecular coils start to overlap and are thus compressed (Fig. 3*a*). This crowding of the chains in this Na-HA matrix increases the chances for various noncovalent chain–chain interactions. This in turn causes considerable increase in the viscosity of the solution. For example, the kinematic viscosity of a 2 mg/ml NaHA (molecular weight 3–4×10^6) in physiologic buffer is only in the magnitude of 100 cSt. At a concentration of 5 mg/ml, the viscosity is in the 10,000 cSt range, and at 10 mg/ml, in the 100,000 cSt range. In other words, a fivefold increase in concentration causes a 1,000-fold increase in the viscosity of the solution. With this increase of viscosity, the elastic properties of the solution also increase (14). The elastic behavior of concentrated (>0.5 mg/ml) NaHA solution is greatly depen-

Na-HYALURONATE
MOLECULAR COILS

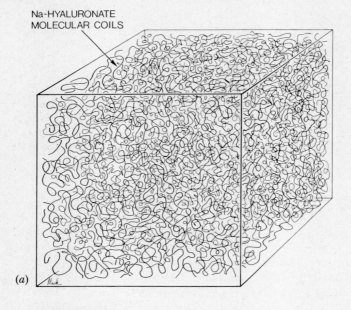

(a)

Na-HYALURONATE
MOLECULAR COILS

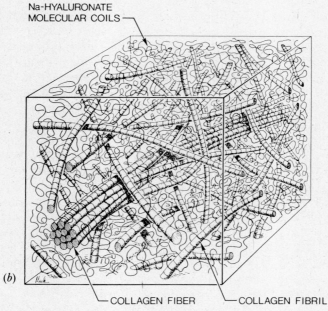

(b)

COLLAGEN FIBER   COLLAGEN FIBRIL

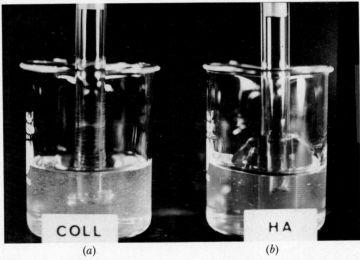

(a)   (b)

Figure 4. The demonstration of viscosity and viscoelasticity in two solutions of biologic macromolecules. (a) 1% solution of tropocollagen dissolved in cold physiologic saline (temp. 5°); (b) 1% sodium hyaluronate dissolved in physiologic saline (temp. 5°). The photograph was taken while the glass tubes were rapidly rotating counterclockwise in the solutions. In the collagen solution (a) a vortex developed, indicating viscosity. The sodium hyaluronate (b) "climbed" both the outside and the inside of the rotating tube. This is the result of the normal stress that occurs in viscoelastic fluids being sheared, and it is called Weissenberg's, or normal, stress effect.

dent on the strain frequency applied to the solution (14); that is, if the mechanical energy is applied to the solution at a low frequency range, the solution responds with viscous flow. On the molecular level, this means that under the imposed strain, the polysaccharide coils slip by each other, and conformational and configurational rearrangements occur while the solution exhibits a viscous flow. At high strain frequencies, this rearrangement cannot occur; thus, the molecular chains deform and the mechanical energy is stored as elasticity. Under these conditions the solution behaves predominantly as an elastic body (Fig. 4). What is unique

←——————————————————————————————————

Figure 3. (a) A three-dimensional model of concentrated (>0.5 mg/ml) sodium hyaluronate solution. (b) A three-dimensional model of concentrated (0.5 mg/ml) sodium hyaluronate solution in which collagen fibrils and fibers (bundle of fibrils) are dispersed. This is also a simplified model of the gel vitreous in such animals as cattle, sheep, owls, and rhesus monkeys and human.

to large molecular weight NaHA molecules dissolved in physiologic buffer is that the transition from the predominantly viscous to predominantly elastic behavior occurs in relatively low concentration (~0.2%) solutions and at a narrow frequency range (0.1–10.0 cycles per second). Since NaHA is present in tissues in this concentration, and biologic systems encounter vibrations of this magnitude, it was proposed that one of the main functions of NaHA in the intercellular matrix is to absorb mechanical stress (15). It has been pointed out that, in such tissues as the vitreous, the cartilage surface of the joint, and the joint capsule, the NaHA alone filling the interfibrillar space of collagen gels is uniquely suited as a shock absorber and structure stabilizer (Fig. 3*b*). Coupled with the load-supporting collagen gel structure, it acts as a reversible mechanical energy-storing and energy-dissipating system (16).

Noninflammatory Fraction of Sodium Hyaluronate (NIF-NaHA, Healon)

It has been shown that sterile, high molecular weight NaHA, after extensive purification to remove proteins, nucleic acids, and other glycosaminoglycans, can still contain a component that causes inflammation when injected into various tissue compartments (6,7,17,18). This inflammation, was characterized as a cellular invasion of nearly exclusively mononuclear cells, mostly macrophages, and is accompanied by increase of the protein concentration that reaches its maximum 48 hours after injection (19). This inflammatory reaction could be quantitated by counting the leukocytes that invaded the tissue compartment where the NaHA was injected. The tissue compartments used were the peritoneal cavity in mice and rats, the joint space in horses, and the liquid vitreous space in owl monkeys and rhesus monkeys (19). While a proper dose–response curve to the inflammatory components in various NaHA solutions could be demonstrated in all three compartments, the vitreous proved to be the most sensitive compartment and yielded the most reproducible results. Thus, in the course of the development of a noninflammatory, high molecular weight NaHA, the owl monkey vitreous test has been used routinely (6,8,19,20).

The owl monkey (*Aotus trivirgatus*) is especially suitable for this test because the relatively large vitreous space (~2 ml) in the adult animal is nearly entirely filled with a viscous liquid vitreous. The viscosity is due to the presence of high molecular weight (~5 × 10^6) NaHA present in the highest concentration observed in any species (0.4–1.0 mg/ml) (21). Approximately half of the viscous liquid vitreous (1 ml) can be removed under sterile surgical conditions with a 25–27G needle and replaced by a sterile test solution without causing major surgical trauma in the eye. The inflammatory reaction caused by the surgical procedure of exchange of the vitreous with the injected substance can be semiquantitatively evaluated by observing the flare and haze in the anterior chamber and vitreous using slit lamp and ophthalmoscope. But, most important, a quantitative assessment of the inflammation in the eye can be made by counting the leukocytes in the aqueous humor. Occasionally, however, the surgical trauma and the injection of the solvent of the NIF-NaHA could cause a reaction of up to 200 cells/mm^3 aqueous humor. Consequently, it became the objective of the developmental work to find a high molecular weight, pure NaHA that did not cause a greater inflammatory reaction in the owl monkey eye than the surgical procedure itself and the replacement of 1 ml liquid vitreous with the same volume of the solvent of the NaHA (8).

In 1976 such a highly purified, large molecular weight NaHA fraction was isolated, and it was called the noninflammatory fraction (NIF) of NaHA (8). Extensive studies were made on owl monkey eyes to evaluate the long-term effect of single or repeated exchanges of the vitreous with the NIF-NaHA (22). Usually 1 ml of a 1% solution of NIF-NaHA (molecular weight 1.2–3 $\times$ 10^6) with a kinematic viscosity of 50–500 $\times$ 10^3 cSt (at 25°C) was used. These studies clearly showed that replacement of the liquid vitreous with NIF-NaHA repeatedly in the same eye as many as nine times did not increase the inflammatory reaction. In other words, the eye did not have any "memory" of previous NIF-NaHA injections. This is extremely important because the possibility of any kind of immunogenicity of the preparation, including possible hypersensitization, is therefore excluded (19).

NIF-NaHA was also used to replace the vitreous in monkeys whose eyes had previously experienced a severe inflammation caused by injection of endotoxin, concanavalin A, or inflammatory NaHA (22). One or two NIF-NaHA injections did not cause any inflammatory reaction, indicating that this substance does not potentiate inflammation initiated by other inflammatory agents. Long-term evaluation (nine years) of monkey eyes in which the vitreous was replaced one to four times showed no pathology except that caused by occasional trauma due to repeated surgical procedures. Histologic and electronmicroscopic studies showed no sign of toxic or immunogenic effects on the retina, lens, or vitreous (22).

NIF-NaHA was first manufactured by Biotrics, Inc. (Arlington, Mass.) and later by Pharmacia AB (Uppsala, Sweden) (8). The only NIF-NaHA available today is called Healon and is manufactured by Pharmacia AB. This preparation contains 10 $\pm$ 1 mg/ml NIF-NaHA dissolved in a physiologic buffer solution (0.146 N NaCl, 0.34 mM NaH_2PO_4, 1.5 mM Na_2HPO_4; pH 7.2 ± 0.2) without any preservative. This solution is sterile and pyrogen-free. The molecular weight of Healon (NIF-NaHA) is 2–4 × 10^6, and the viscosity of the solution is 100–300 × 10^3 cSt.

The amino acid content of Healon is <0.03%, and the impurity of other glycosaminoglycans is <0.2% of the NaHA content. Healon did not show any immunogenicity when tested either by the monkey eye test (19,22) or by passive cutaneous anaphylaxis tests in rabbits and humans (23,24).

SODIUM HYALURONATE IN THE ANTERIOR CHAMBER

Passage Time

In the human aqueous humor the NaHA concentration is only one-hundredth that of vitreous (11,13). This very small amount (1–3 μg/ml) originates from the vitreous via a posterior chamber (25,26). It is also possible that the corneal endothelial cells may contribute a small amount. When in monkey eyes (owl monkey or rhesus monkey) part of the liquid vitreous is replaced with NIF-NaHA solution (10 μg/ml), the concentration of NaHA in the anterior chamber increases rapidly and remains above normal level as long as the concentration in the vitreous remains elevated (25,26,27). The molecular size of the NIF-NaHA injected into the vitreous is unchanged as it passes to the anterior chamber.

When NIF-NaHA is injected into the anterior chamber of the owl monkey eye, its residence time depends on the amount injected and on the viscosity of the solution. Extensive studies were carried out on the primate eye using six samples of different viscosities (940, 291, 236, 106, 41, and 10 × 10^3 cSt) of the same concentration (10 mg/ml) NIF-NaHA solution (28,29). Two different volumes (0.22 and 0.35 ml) were used to replace some of the aqueous humor representing approximately 50% and 75% respectively of the total aqueous humor volume in this animal. When the smaller volume was injected, the rate of disappearance depended entirely on the viscosity. The highest viscosity sample cleared the anterior chamber with a rate of 50 μl/h aqueous flow and the lowest with 120 μl/h. The rates of clearance of the rest of the samples were between these two values. This means that 24 hours after the injection 27% of the 940,000 cSt sample remained in the anterior chamber, but during this same time all of the 10,000 cSt sample was washed out by the fast-flowing aqueous humor. When a larger volume of the aqueous humor was replaced, it took, as would be expected, a longer time for the NIF-NaHA to clear the anterior chamber. But most important the initial rate of disappearance was much slower. The aqueous flow was 30 μl/h for the highest and 70 μl/h for the lowest viscosity samples. After the first 24 hours 50% of the highest viscosity and 15% of the lowest

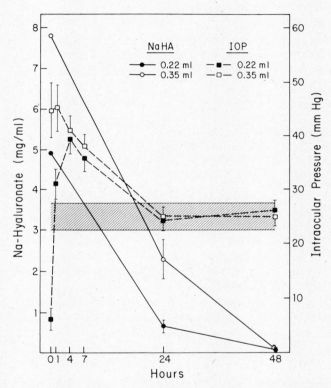

Figure 5. Sodium hyaluronate concentration in the anterior chamber and IOP in the owl monkey eye at various times after partial replacement of the aqueous humor with 1% sterile solution of NIF-NaHA. 0.22 ml aqueous humor was removed and replaced by 0.22 or 0.35 ml of NIF-NaHA solution, which had a kinematic viscosity of 106,000 cSt. This represented a 50% or 75% replacement of the aqueous humor with the NIF-NaHA solution. It also created an "under-filled" (0.22 ml) or "overfilled" (0.35 ml) anterior chamber with an initially lower or higher than normal IOP. The shaded area indicates the normal range IOP. The concentration of NaHA in the normal aqueous humor of the owl monkey is 0.0056 ± 0.0008 mg/ml. (This figure represents data taken from the work of Schubert, Denlinger, and Balazs, 1981: ref. 29.)

viscosity sample remained in the anterior chamber. The lowest viscosity samples completely cleared the anterior chamber within 48 hours after injection. But three days after injection, 11% of the highest viscosity sample still remained, and only during the fourth day did all of it disappear from the anterior chamber.

In the owl monkey eye the medium viscosity samples clear the anterior chamber in 48 hours if only 50% of the aqueous humor is replaced, and within 72 hours if 75% is replaced (Fig. 5).

The molecular size of the NIF-NaHA injected into the owl monkey anterior chamber does not change significantly during its residence there. This means that extracellular degrading enzymes or oxidative agents are not present. Thus, the NaHA most likely passes through the trabecular tissue as a large, voluminous molecule. It is, however, still much smaller than the blood cells and the particles originating from the zonular fibers and postoperative fibrin precipitates in the anterior chamber. Thus, in the outflow channels in the living eye, unlike those in the enucleated eye, viscous fluid with suspended particles can pass through the angle because in the living eye the angle is in a dynamic state. There is constant movement owing to the contraction of the ciliary muscles and to the contractile elements of the cells of the trabecular system. Therefore, viscous solutions and particles do not simply pass through, but rather are moved through the system.

The NaHA from Schlemm's canal passes to the blood where it is quickly picked up by the liver. Here most likely the Kupffer cells are responsible for the pinocytosis and degradation of the NaHA by lysosomal enzymes. NaHA in the blood is present in a very low concentration (in humans 0.15–0.55 μg/ml) originating mainly from the lymph, which in turn collects it from the connective tissue matrices (30,73).

Effect on the Intraocular Pressure

When viscous solutions of NIF-NaHA are injected into the anterior chamber of rabbit and owl monkey eyes, a temporary increase in the IOP can be observed only when the concentration at any time after the injection is greater than 2 mg NaHA per 1 ml aqueous humor (Fig. 5). Since in these animals the normal NaHA concentration in the aqueous humor is 0.0005–0.005 mg/ml, this represents a 400- to 4,000-fold increase.

Extensive studies were carried out on owl monkeys (31) and rabbits (32) to establish the effect on IOP of exogenous, viscous NIF-NaHA solutions injected into the anterior chamber. When viscous (100,000–200,000 cSt) solutions of 10 mg/ml NaHA were injected into the anterior chamber causing an immediate 5,000- to 20,000-fold increase over the normal NaHA concentration, the IOP peaked in three to four hours and returned to normal in 24 hours. The cornea, lens, and anterior chamber remained as clear as in the control animals in which the physiologic buffer solvent of the NaHA solution was injected.

Recently, a more comprehensive study was made on owl monkey eyes to investigate the effect of the viscosity of the NaHA solution on the postoperative IOP (28,29). NIF-NaHA (Healon) was injected in 10 mg/ml concentrations, and the viscosity of the solutions was varied between 10,000 and 940,000 cSt. These differences in viscosity were controlled by altering the molecular weight ($1.3–4.9 \times 10^6$) and molecular interaction. The immediate postinjection IOP was adjusted to lower than normal (8–12 mm Hg) and higher than normal (40–50 mm Hg) levels by replacing 0.22 ml aqueous humor by equal volume (low pressure group) or by the greater volume of NIF-NaHA (0.35 ml, high pressure group). When the immediate postinjection pressure was kept below 12 mm Hg with solutions of viscosity greater than 230,000 cSt, no significant increase in the IOP was noted during the 72-hour postoperative period (Fig. 5). When the immediate postinjection pressure was kept below 12 mm Hg with 41,000 and 108,000 cSt samples, the IOP rose significantly above 12 mm Hg between four to seven hours, but reached normal levels 24 hours after injection. When the immediate postinjection pressure was kept below 12 mm Hg with the lowest viscosity sample (10,000 cSt), intraocular pressures reaching 60 mm Hg were noted seven hours postinjection. Twenty-four hours after injection the IOP in these eyes also returned to a normal level.

In those cases where the IOP was adjusted above normal, every viscosity caused a substantial increase in the pressure, reaching a maximum level four hours postinjection. The sample with 108,000 cSt viscosity showed a significantly lower level IOP (40 ± 10 mm Hg) than the rest of the samples (60 ± 10 mm Hg). In all cases, the IOP returned to normal 24 hours later and remained normal. In all these experiments the NaHA concentration in the anterior chamber was measured at various times. It was found that the IOP, even if it was temporarily elevated, returned to normal even though the concentration of the injected NIF-NaHA still was as high as 1–3 mg/ml.

It is interesting to note that injection of the lowest viscosity sample resulted in the highest IOP. This can be explained by the fact that the high viscosity NIF-NaHA solutions are more coherent; in other words, they are more difficult to dilute. That is, the newly formed aqueous humor can only wash away the highly viscous jelly very slowly. Therefore, during the first hours, the aqueous humor reaching the outflow channels has low NaHA concentration and therefore it is not very viscous, causing no slowdown in flow and consequently no elevation in IOP. However, the low viscosity sample quickly mixes with the newly formed aqueous humor. Thus, the outflowing aqueous humor is very viscous in the beginning, and its flow through the outflow channels is slow, causing an elevation of IOP.

These studies clearly show that in experimental animals, when the normal eye is minimally traumatized, the injection of even the most viscous NIF-NaHA solution, which is 940,000 times more viscous than the aqueous humor, causes only a transient increase in IOP, which then returns to normal levels in 24 hours. If the injected 10 mg/ml NIF-NaHA solution replaces less than half of the aqueous humor volume, the IOP does not increase significantly at all.

The human clinical situation after anterior segment surgery is naturally more complicated than in the animal experiments described above. First of all, the larger incision may traumatize part of the trabecular tissue. The closer the incision is to the limbus, the greater the trauma. For example, corneal incisions are less apt to cause elevation of IOP postoperatively because they are farther from the trabecular meshwork.

Second, inflammation caused by traumatizing iris, corneal endothelium, ciliary body, lens capsule, and epithelium and zonules may produce an exudate that fills the anterior chamber. This exudate contains living and dead cells and cell debris from the neighboring tissues. If an intracapsular lens extraction is performed with α-chymotrypsin, the anterior chamber would also contain segments of the zonular fibers. Thus, all the effects described tend to make the human clinical situation different from the animal experiments described previously.

SODIUM HYALURONATE IN THE VITREOUS

Extensive studies were carried out in monkeys (owl monkey and rhesus monkey) to determine the exit path and the residence time of NIF-NaHA in the vitreous (20,25,26,27). Both species of monkey have a large volume of liquid vitreous. Thus a viscoelastic solution of the NIF-NaHA can replace an equal volume of liquid vitreous with minimal postoperative inflammation. In the owl monkey, half ot the injected NaHA diffuses out through the anterior face of the vitreous gel in approximately 63 days, and all is gone in 120 days. In these experiments the rate of passage depends upon the integrity of the anterior cortical gel (25,33,67), which is very thin and easily damaged during the vitreous exchange operation. If the anterior cortical gel is damaged, the injected NaHA will quickly pass into the posterior chamber, and within three to six days the injected NaHA will disappear from the vitreous. This observation emphasizes the importance of the structure of the anterior cortical vitreous gel as a diffusion barrier and the size of the annular gap between ciliary processes and the lens as the controlling factors of the NaHA content of the vitreous. It has also been noted that after intracapsular lens extraction in both monkeys and in humans, the NaHA concentration in the vitreous falls below normal (68,69). This was explained by the fact that after the lens and its capsule are removed, the vitreal NaHA can pass directly into the anterior chamber. The exit opening is larger, and therefore the steady state concentration of NaHA in the vitreous becomes lower.

These monkey studies also suggest that the residence time of NaHA in the vitreous will depend on such factors as the concentration, viscosity, and volume of the NaHA solution exchanged with the vitreous; the thickness, the density, and the structural integrity of the anterior cortical gel; the presence or absence of the lens capsule (which is impermeable to the large NaHA molecules); and, finally, the extent of the inflammatory process present in the vitreous. Specifically, the residence time of the injected NaHA will be the longest when a large volume of concentrated, high viscous NIF-NaHA solution is injected without damaging the anterior cortical gel into a phakic eye with very little postoperative inflammation and no hemorrhage. A strong postoperative inflammation, without hemorrhage, makes the injected NaHA residence time shorter because many of the invading inflammatory cells (macrophages) will remove the NaHA by pinocytosis. Intravitreal hemorrhage also can shorten the residence time. During red cell cytolysis, substances are released that cause degradation of the large NaHA molecules into smaller molecules that can then diffuse faster through the anterior cortical gel.

THE CONCEPT OF VISCOSURGERY

The word "viscosurgery" was coined by tbe author (34) to indicate procedures in which viscoelastic solutions or pastes are used to protect cells from mechanical trauma, to maintain or create tissue spaces, to ensure separation and lubrication of tissue surfaces, to permit the manipulation of tissues without mechanical damage, and to prevent and control movement and activities of certain cells.

Cell Protection

Epithelial cells constantly exposed to mechanical trauma, such as mucous membranes, are protected by heavy glycoprotein layers (mucous secretion). If they are destroyed mechanically, chemically, or by heat damage, they rapidly regenerate. Fibrocytes, smooth muscle cells, and histiocytes of the connective tissues are embedded in viscoelastic, extracellular matrices that serve to protect them from the mechanical trauma of the constant deformation of the tissues. Endothelial and epithelial cells that are normally not exposed to mechanical trauma, such as corneal and trabecular endothelium, lens, and ciliary epithelium, are unprotected. Furthermore, often they do not possess regenerative potential (corneal endothelium). During surgical manipulation and in course of introduction of solid implants, these cells are exposed to considerable mechanical damage; therefore, the introduction of viscoelastic solutions or jellies into these usually protected areas provide a physiologic type of protection (57–61,63).

Viscoelastic solutions can be used to protect epithelial tissue such as the corneal epithelium from mechanical damage and from drying out. Viscous NaHA solutions were used as tear substitutes, either when the secretion was impaired (dry eye) (72) or when the muscular paralysis prevented or decreased the frequency of blinking. In these cases the viscoelastic solution acted as a protective layer against mechanical or chemical damage caused by the dry lid or by dust particles and microorganisms. The water that fills the intramolecular domain of NaHA evaporates only slowly, and therefore the corneal surface remains covered by the hydrated NaHA layer for a long time. While the mechanism of protection and hydration of the epithelium is not the same as that of the natural tear layer, the viscous NaHA solutions were well tolerated by extremely dry eyes and clinically were very effective.

Maintenance of Tissue Spaces

Tissue spaces filled with liquids (aqueous humor, liquid vitreous, synovial fluid, cerebrospinal fluid) often collapse partially or completely during surgical procedures. Viscoelastic solutions and pastes can conveniently maintain these spaces even when a considerable opening is created during surgery. The cohesive nature of the viscoelastic pastes makes them flow very slowly, and therefore they remain in place after their introduction for a considerable time. When a new tissue space must be created, such as the subconjunctival space in glaucoma surgery, or an existing narrow space has to be extended, such as in some tendon surgery, a viscoelastic solution or paste can achieve this goal without capillary trauma and subsequent hemorrhage or exudation (36,62).

Tissue Lubrication

Permanent separation of internal tissue surfaces is maintained normally by two structural systems. Two surface epithelia may be separated by a viscous glycoprotein or glycosaminoglycan secretion, as is found in the peritoneal, pericardial, and pleural spaces. The second case involves the separation of connective tissue surfaces. Typical examples are the liquid vitreous, the joint space, the space between tendon and tendon sheaths, and the subcutaneous tissue and fascia-covered spaces. In all these cases, natural NaHA plays a very important role, both in filling the interfibrillar spaces of the collagen gel matrix and separating the collagen matrices.

The major biologic role of NaHA is to lubricate collagen gel surfaces. Lubrication, in this context, means the protection of the solid collagen gel surfaces from dislocation (14). The surface layers of the collagen gel imbibed with and covered by the viscoelastic NaHA are protected from mechanical stress. So are the cells embedded in the very superficial layers of this collagen gel. When natural or surgical trauma (inflammation, hemorrhage) disrupts these two types of compartments, adhesions based on the fibrin coagulum form that are later organized into collagen fibrous scar tissue. Viscoelastic solutions or pastes of NaHA can be used to separate surfaces already immobilized by adhesions. This was found to be useful in treatment of joint stiffness caused by capsular adhesions. These solutions and pastes can also prevent adhesion formation when applied after surgery between tendons and tendon sheaths (35,36,37). When it is injected intraarticularly, it can improve loss of joint function that occurs as a consequence of traumatic arthritis or joint immobilization (38–42).

Tissue Manipulation

The first use of viscoelastic pastes of NaHA in conjunction with eye surgery was conceived in order to be able to manipulate the detached retina without touching it with instruments (4,31). Viscoelastic solutions and pastes were used to push back the retina to its desired anatomic position and retain the retina in this position. Unlike gases and physiologic saline solution also used for this purpose, the viscoelastic paste does not pass through the holes and breaks of the retina into the subretinal space. This internal tamponade concept works best when the viscoelastic paste is placed inside of the gel vitreous or into a liquid vitreous pocket separated from the retina by the cortical vitreous gel. In both cases, when the volume of the internal tamponade is expanded, it pushes against the gel vitreous, which in turn pushes back the retina (50–56,71).

The viscoelastic solution can also be used for the manipulation of the anterior face of the vitreous gel as an external tamponade. It was found that in the aphakic eye the forward bulge of the weakened, but not yet broken, anterior cortical vitreous gel can be controlled by the viscoelastic solutions. This coherent viscoelastic external tamponade wedged between the cornea and iris can exert a considerable pressure on the anterior vitreous gel and push it back. This is hard to achieve with instruments because of the adhesion between collagen fibers and the instrument, which tends to tear the vitreous face (63).

Manipulation of tissues in a space filled with viscoelastic solution can provide other advantages (43,74). The movement of tissue is damped by the viscoelastic solution, and the manipulation of tissues under the operating microscope can be facilitated. Bleeding caused by the surgical manipulation can be restricted to a small area because the blood cells cannot spread into the viscoelastic solution and therefore are kept in the immediate vicinity of the vessel damage.

Control of Cell Activity

Viscous media inhibit the cell membrane activity of the cells of the reticuloendothelial and lymphatic systems. This was first demonstrated with viscoelastic solutions of NaHA and NIF-NaHA. These solutions inhibit the in vitro migration of granulocytes, macrophages, and peripheral and blood lymphocytes (44). The phagocytic activity of macrophages and granulocytes is also completely inhibited as is the synthesis and release of prostaglandins by macrophages during phagocytosis (45,46). The transformation of lymphocytes to lymphoblasts and the subsequent cell division is inhibited by viscous NaHA solutions (47) and liquid vitreous (70). Similarly, the in vitro growth of vascular endothelial cells, which are also part of the reticuloendothelial system, is inhibited (48). All this inhibitory function is not due to the chemical characteristics of the NaHA molecule, but rather to the rheological properties of the solution. It was demonstrated that viscous solutions of proteins (gelatin) and nucleic acids (DNA) have the same effect (49). On the other hand, nonviscous solution of other stronger polyanions, such as heparin or chondroitin sulfates, in similar or even higher concentration do not have any such effects (45).

Thus an additional dimension is added to the viscosurgical use of NIF-NaHA. The viscoelastic solution remaining after surgery slows down or completely prevents the invasion, activity, and proliferation of the inflammatory cells and the release of some inflammatory mediators. This means that the viscous solutions of NIF-NaHA have some anti-inflammatory characteristics. This could be the reason NIF-NaHA prevents postoperative adhesion formation and cellular infiltration. Interestingly, NIF-NaHA solutions do not inhibit the movements of fibroblasts and epithelial cells and consequently do not interfere with wound healing and reepithelialization.

CONCLUSION

Viscosurgery or the application of viscoelastic devices can be carried out only with substances that fulfill several important criteria. First of all, the substance must be biologically inert. In addition, they must be nontoxic, sterile, and pyrogen-free. The definition of biologic inertness is a complex one. It excludes substances that cause formation of antibodies (protein, glycoproteins, proteoglycans). Also eliminated are substances causing granulation tissue formation (all plant polysaccharides) and connective tissue encapsulation (organic polymers, silicon substances, etc.) Substances that stimulate local inflammation (NaHA) or interfere with blood coagulation, epithelialization, and endothelialization (sulfated glycosaminoglycans) cannot be regarded as biologically inert substances. In addition, the biologically suitable substance must remain at the surgical location long enough to exert its effect. Therefore substances that are very rapidly biodegraded are not usable (nucleic acids).

In addition to these negative characteristics the ideal substance must be extremely viscoelastic at a relatively low concentration when dissolved in a physiologically balanced salt solution. Somewhat viscoelastic solutions can be made from concentrated solutions (5%) of sulfated glycosaminoglycans such as chondroitin sulfates. But in this concentration the polyanionic solutions will exert strong general antienzyme and osmotic activities, which is not desirable. Another advantage in achieving high viscosity and elasticity at low concentration of the material used is the high water content of the viscosurgical or viscomedical device. That is, if the solution or paste contains 1% salt and 1–3% of the polymer, the water content will be 97–98%. This permits the free, unaltered diffusion of all metabolites to and from the cells, which is extremely important especially when large intercellular tissue compartments like the vitreous space or the anterior chamber are filled.

The elastic nature of the material is not only important in acting as a "shock absorber" and providing structural stabilization, but also for facilitating the passage of the viscous solution through small channels. When the viscosity of a nonelastic solution is over 10,000 cSt, it can be pushed through a small opening only with great force. If a fluid has elastic as well as viscous properties, that can mean, but not necessarily, that the individual molecular coils are deformable. Such a deformable coil system can be pushed through small orifices (such as a 28G needle) even when the viscosity is extremely high (>100,000 cSt).

Today, the only substance known that fulfills the above criteria is the NIF-NaHA. This biopolymer has the additional advantage that it is the natural shock absorber, structure stabilizer, and space separator in the vertebrate body. When applied as a therapeutic device, it is nearly always used at locations where normally it is present but in a lower concentration. Thus its therapeutic effectiveness and the remarkable lack of side effects can be attributed to the fact that its use simply creates a temporary increase of the concentration in an extracellular matrix where NaHA is a biologically important component.

REFERENCES

1. Balazs, E.A. *The Interaction of Chemical and Mechanical Factors in Bone Regeneration,* thesis, Univ. Budapest, Fac. Med, 1942.

2. Balazs, E.A., Piller, L. The formation of the synovial fluid. *Magy. Orv. Arch.* 44:3, 1943.

3. Meyer, K., Smyth, E.M., Dawson, M.H. The isolation for a mucopolysaccharide from synovial fluid. *J. Biol. Chem.* 128:319–327, 1936.

4. Balazs, E.A. Physiology of the vitreous body, in Schepens, C.L. (ed): *Importance of the Vitreous Body in Retina Surgery with Special Emphasis on Reoperations.* St. Louis, Mosby, 1960, pp. 29–48, 144–146.

5. Balazs, E.A., Sweeney, D.B. The use of hyaluronic acid and collagen preparations in eye surgery, in Schepens, C.L., Regan, C.D.J. (eds): *Controversial Aspects of the Management of Retinal Detachment.* Boston, Little, Brown, 1965, pp. 200–202.

6. Balazs, E.A., Sweeney, D.B. Replacement of the vitreous body of monkeys with reconstituted vitreous and hyaluronic acid, in Streiff, E.B. (ed): *Modern Problems in Ophthalmology (Surgery of Retinal Vascular Diseases and Prophylactic Treatment of Retinal Detachment, Amersfoort, 1963).* Basel, Karger, 1966, pp. 230–232.

7. Balazs, E.A., Sweeney, D.B. The injection of hyaluronic acid and reconstituted vitreous into the vitreous cavity, in McPherson, A. (ed): *New and Controversial Aspects of Retinal Detachment.* New York, Harper & Row, 1968, pp. 371–376.

8. Balazs, E.A. Ultrapure hyaluronic acid and the use thereof. U.S. Patent No. 4.141.973, 1979.

9. Balazs, E.A. Hyaluronic Acid and Matrix Implantation. Arlington, Mass, Biotrics, Inc., 1971.

10. Comper, W.D., Laurent, T.C. Physiological function of connective tissue polysaccharides. *Physiol. Rev.* 58:255–315, 1978.

11. Balazs, E.A. Amino sugar-containing macromolecules in the tissues of the eye and the ear, in Balazs, E.A., Jeanloz, R.W. (eds): *The Amino Sugars: The Chemistry and Biology of Compounds Containing Amino Sugars. II-A. Distribution and Biological Role.* New York, Academic Press, 1965, pp. 401–460.

12. Denlinger, J.L., Eisner, G., Balazs, E.A. Age-related changes in the vitreous and lens of rhesus monkeys (*Macaca* mulatta): I. Initial biomicroscopic and biochemical survey of free-ranging animals. *Exp. Eye Res.* 31:67–69, 1980.

13. Laurent, U.B.G. Hyaluronate in aqueous humor. *Exp. Eye Res.* 33:147–155, 1981.

14. Balazs, E.A., Gibbs, D.A. The rheological properties and biological function of hyaluronic acid, in Balazs, E.A. (ed): *Chemistry and Molecular Biology of the Intercellular Matrix.* New York, Academic Press, 1970, pp. 1241–1254.

15. Balazs, E.A. Viscoelastic properties of hyaluronic acid and biological lubrication. (Symposium: Prognosis for Arthritis: Rheumatology Research Today and Prospects for Tomorrow, Ann Arbor, Michigan, 1967). *Univ. Mich. Med. Ctr. J.*, suppl., 1968, pp. 255–259.

16. Balazs, E.A. Some aspects of the aging and radiation sensitivity of the intercellular matrix with special regard to hyaluronic acid in synovial fluid and vitreous, in Engel, A., Larsson, T. (eds): *Thule International Symposium: Aging of Connective and Skeletal Tissue.* Stockholm, Nordiska Bokhandelns Förlag, 1969, pp. 107–122.

17. Constable, I.J., Swann, D.A. Biological vitreous substitutes: Inflammatory response in normal and altered animal eyes. *Arch. Ophthalmol.* 88:544–548, 1972.

18. Swann, DA Studies on hyaluronic acid: I. The preparation and properties of rooster comb hyaluronic acid. *Biochim Biophys. Acta* 156:17–30, 1968.

19. Denlinger, J.L., Balazs, E.A. Replacement of the liquid vitreus with sodium hyaluronate in monkeys: I. Short term evaluation. *Exp. Eye Res.* 31:81–99, 1980.

20. Balazs, E.A., Hultsch, E. Replacement of the vitreous with hyaluronic acid, collagen and other polymers, in Irvine, A.R., O'Malley, C. (eds): *Advances in Vitreous Surgery.* Springfield, Il, Charles C Thomas, 1976.

21. Österlinn, S.E., Balazs, E.A. Macromolecular composition and fine structure of the vitreous in the owl monkey. *Exp. Eye Res.* 7:534–545, 1968.

22. Denlinger, J.L., El-Mofty, A.M., Balazs, E.A. Replacement of the liquid vitreus with sodium hyaluronate in monkeys: II. Long term evaluation. *Exp. Eye Res.* 31:101–117, 1980.

23. Richter, A.W. Non-immunogenicity of purified hyaluronic acid preparations tested by passive cutaneous anaphylaxis. *Int. Arch. Allergy Appl. Immunol.* 47:211–217, 1974.

24. Richter, A.W., Ryde, E.M., Zetterstrom, E.O. Non-immunogenicity of a purified sodium hyaluronate preparation in man. *Int. Arch. Allergy Appl. Immunol.* 59:45–48, 1979.

25. Balazs, E.A., Freeman, M.I., Regnault, F. The fate of hyaluronic acid injected into the vitreous of owl monkey, in Balazs, E.A.: *Hyaluronic Acid and Matrix Implantation.* Arlington, Mass, Biotrics, Inc., 1971.

26. Denlinger, J.L., Balazs, E.A., Flood, M.T., Forrester, J.V. Age-related changes of the vitreous of the rhesus monkey and the metabolism of hyaluronic acid, abstracted. Third International Congress of Eye Research, Osaka, Japan, 1978.

27. Denlinger, J.L., Balazs, E.A., Flood, M.T., Forrester, J.V. Metabolism of hyaluronic acid in monkey vitreus: II. Transport rate. (In press)

28. Denlinger, J.L., Schubert, H., Balazs, E.A. Na-hyaluronate of various molecular sizes injected into the anterior chamber of owl monkey; disappearance and effect on intraocular pressure. *Proc. Int. Soc. Eye Res.* 1:88, 1980.

29. Schubert, H., Denlinger, J.L., and Balazs, E.A. Na-hyaluronate injected into the anterior chamber of the owl monkey: Effect on iop and rate of disappearance. *Invest. Ophthalmol. Vis. Sci.* 20(suppl):118, 1981.

30. Laurent, U.B.G., Laurent, T.C. On the origin of hyaluronate in blood. *Biochem. Int.* 2:195–199, 1981.

31. Balazs, E.A., Freeman, M.I., Klöti, R. Meyer-Schwickerath, G., Regnault, F., Sweeney, D.B. Hyaluronic acid and replacement of vitreous and aqueous humor. *Mod. Probl. Ophthalmol.* 10:3–21, 1972.

32. Miller, D., O'Connor, P., Williams, J. Use of Na-hyaluronate during intraocular lens implantation in rabbits. *Ophthalmic Surg.* 8:58061, 1977.

33. Denlinger, J.L., El-Mofty, A.A.M., Balazs, E.A. Metabolism of hyaluronic acid in monkey vitreus: VI. Role of the anterior cortical vitreous gel. (In press)

34. Balazs, E.A., Miller, D., Stegmann, R. Viscosurgery and the use of Na-hyaluronate in intraocular lens implantation. Paper presented at the International Congress and First Film Festival on Intraocular Implantation, Cannes, France, 1979.

35. Rydell, N., Balazs, E.A. Effect of intra-articular injection of hyaluronic acid on the clinical symptoms of osteoarthritis and on granulation tissue formation. *Clin. Orthop.* 80:25–32, 1971.

36. St. Onge, R., Weiss, C., Denlinger, J.L., Balazs, E.A. A preliminary clinical assessment of Na-hyaluronate injection for primary flexor tendon repair in no-man's land. *Clin. Orthop.* 146:269–275, 1980.

37. Rydell, N. Decreased granulation tissue reaction after installment of hyaluronic acid. *Acta Orthop. Scand.* 307–311, 1970.

38. Rydell, N.W., Butler, J., Balazs, E.A. Hyaluronic acid in synovial fluid: VI. Effect of intra-articular injection of hyaluronic acid on the clinical symptoms of arthritis in track horses. *Acta Vet. Scand.* 11:139–155, 1970.

39. Peyron, J.G., Balazs, E.A. Preliminary clinical assessment of Na-hyaluronate injection into human arthritic joints. *Pathol. Biol.* 22:732–736, 1974.

40. Balazs, E.A. The physical properties of synovial fluid and the special role of hyaluronic acid, in Helfet, A. (ed): *Disorders of the Knee.* Philadelphia, J.B. Lippincott, 1974, pp. 63–75.

41. Äsheim, Ä., Lindblad, G. Intra-articular treatment of arthritis in race-horses with sodium hyaluronate. *Acta Vet. Scand.* 17:379–394, 1976.

42. Weiss, C., Balazs, E.A., St. Onge, R., Denlinger, J.L. Clinical studies of the intraarticular injection of Healon® (sodium hyaluronate) in the treatment of osteoarthritis of human knees, in Talbott, J.H. (ed): *Seminars in Arthr. and Rheu.* New York, Grune & Stratton, 1981, chap. 11.

43. Pruett, R.C., Schepens, C.L., Constable, I.J. et al. Hyaluronic acid vitreous substitute, in Freeman H.M., Hirose T., Schepens C.L. (eds): *Vitreous Surgery and Advances in Fundus Diagnosis and Treatment.* New York, Appleton-Century-Crofts, 1977, pp. 433–443.

44. Balazs, E.A., Darzynkiewewicz, Z. The effect of hyaluronic acid on fibroplasts, mononuclear phagocytes and lymphocytes. (Papers of the symposium held in Turku, Finland, 1972.) Kulonen, E., Pikkarainen, J. (eds): *Biology of the Fibroblast.* New York, Academic Press, 1973, vol. I, p. 237.

45. Forrester, J.V., Balazs, E.A. Inhibition of phagocytosis by high molecular weight hyaluronate. *Immunology* 40:435–446, 1980.

46. Sebag, J., Balazs, E.A., Eakins, K.E., et al. The effect of hyaluronic acid on prostaglandin synthesis and phagocytosis by mononuclear phagocytes *in vitro.* (In press)

47. Darzynkiewicz, Z., Balazs, E.A. Effect of connective tissue intercellular matrix on lymphocyte stimulation: I. Suppression of lymphocyte stimulation by hyaluronic acid. *Exp. Cell Res.* 66:113–123, 1971.

48. Raymond, L., Jacobson, B. Isolation and inhibitory cell growth factors in bovine vitreous. *Exp. Eye Res.,* 1981. (In press)

49. Balazs, E.A. Unpublished data.

50. Algvere, P. Intravitreal implantation of a high-molecular hyaluronic acid in surgery for retinal detachment. *Acta Ophthalmol* 49:975–976, 1971.

51. Regnault, F. Acide hyaluronique intravitréen et cryocoagulation dans le traitement des formes graves de décollement de la rétine. *Bull. Soc. Ophthalmol. Fr.,* 1971.

52. Klöti, R. Hyaluronsäure als Glaskörpersubstituent. *Schweiz. Ophthal. Ges.* 165:351–359, 1972.

53. Edmund, J. Vitreous substitute in the treatment of retinal detachment. Limitations and prospects for retinal surgery. *Mod. Probl. Ophthalmol.* 12:370–377, 1974.

54. Regnault, F., Bregeat, P. Treatment of severe cases of retinal detachment with highly viscous hyaluronic acid. Limitatins and prospects for retinal surgery. *Mod. Probl. Ophthalmol.* 12:378–383, 1974.

55. Kanski, J.J. Intravitreal hyaluronic acid injection. A long-term clinical evaluation. *Br. J. Ophthalmol.* 59:255, 1975.

56. Schepens, C.L., Constable, I.J. Open-sky vitrectomy: Operative technique and instrumentation, in Freeman H.M., Hirose T., Schepens C.L. (eds): *Vitreous Surgery and Advances in Fundus Diagnosis and Treatment.* New York, Appleton-Century-Crofts, 1977, pp. 465–467.

57. Edmund, J. Comments on the clinical use of Healon and a short survey of the use of intraocular injection of hyaluronic acid, in Irvine, O'Malley (eds): *Advances in Vitreus Surgery.* Springfield, Il., Charles C Thomas, 1976, pp. 624–625.

58. Miller, D., Stegmann, R. Use of sodium hyaluronate in anterior segment eye surgery. *Am. Intraocular Implant Soc. J.* 6:13–15, 1980.

59. Miller, D., Stegmann, R. Use of Na-hyaluronate in auto-corneal transplantation in rabbits. *Opthalmic Surg.* 11:19–21, 1980.

60. Stanifer, R., Kretzer, F., Mesta, R. Effect of Healon on intraocular pressure, corneal thickness, and endothelial morphology in the rabbit. *Invest. Ophthalmol. Vis. Sci.* 20:230, 1981.

61. Graue, E.L., Polack, F.M., Balazs, E.A. The protective effect of Na-hyaluronate to corneal endothelium *Exp. Eye Res.* 31:119–127, 1979.

62. Pape, L.G., Balazs, E.A. The use of sodium hyaluronate (Healon®) in human anterior segment surgery. *Ophthalmology* 87:699–705, 1980.

63. Polack, F.M., Balazs, E.A., Miller, D., et al. Viscosurgery of anterior segment. 1980 instruction section course 301. *Am. Acad. Ophthalmol.*, 1980.

64. Balazs, E.A., Armand, G. Glycosaminoglycans and proteoglycans of ocular tissues, in Varmas, R. (ed): *Glycosaminoglycans and Proteoglycans in Physiological and Pathological Processes of Body Systems.* Basel, Karger, 1982, (in press).

65. Barany, E.H. The action of different kinds of hyaluronidase on the resistance to flow through the angle of the anterior chamber. *Acta Ophthalmol.* 34:397–403, 1956.

66. Berson, F.G., Epstein, D.L., Patterson, M.M. Obstruction of outflow facility by sodium hyaluronate in post-mortem enucleated human eyes. *Invest. Ophthalmol. Vis. Sci.* 20:119, 1981.

67. Hultsch, E., Balazs, E.A. Transport of hyaluronic acid from vitreous: Mechanism and dynamics. Annual Meeting of the Association for Research in Vision and Ophthalmology (ARVO), 1975, p. 2.

68. Österlin, S. Macromolecular composition of the vitreous in the aphakic owl monkey eye. *Exp. Eye Res.* 26:77–84, 1978.

69. Österlin, S. On the molecular biology of the vitreous in the aphakic eye. *Acta Ophthalmol.* 55:353–361, 1977.

70. Hultsch, E., Darzynkiewicz, Z., Balazs, E.A. Suppression of lymphocyte-lymphoblast transformation by the vitreous and its macromolecular components. ARVO Abstr, Sarasota, 24.

71. Girod, P., Rouchy, J.P. L'acide hyaluronique dans la chirurgie du corps vitré. Reflexion à propos de 24 cas. *Ann. Ocul.* 203:25, 1970.

72. Polack, F.M., Balazs, E.A., McNiece, M. The use of sodium hyaluronate (Healon®) in the treatment of keratitis sicra. Scientific poster. Academy of Ophthalmology Meeting, Atlanta, Ga, Nov. 1981.

73. Fraser, J.R.E., Laurent, T.C., Pertoft, H., Baxter, E. Plasma clearance, tissue distribution and metabolism of hyaluronic acid injected intravenously in the rabbit. *Biochem. J.* 200:415–424, 1981.

74. Pruett, R.C., Schepens, C.L., Swann, D.A. Hyaluronic acid vitreous substitute. A six-year clinical evaluation. *Arch. Ophthalmol.* 97:2325–2330, 1979.

75. Laurent, U.B.G., Granath, K.A. The molecular weight of hyaluronate in the aqueous humor and vitreous body of rabbit and cattle eyes. Personal communication, 1982.

76. Balazs, E.A., and Denlinger, J.L. Vitreous and joint: Comparative morphology and biochemistry. Fondazione Giorgio Ronchi, Capri, Italy. *Centro di Studio e di Vita, Italy Atti Della Fondazione Giorgio Ronchi* 34:637–647, 1979.

2

Intracapsular Cataract Extraction with Healon

Robert Stegmann

David Miller

INTRODUCTION

The history of the development of the intracapsular cataract extraction is dotted with many milestones. In 1753, Dr. Samuel Sharp of London performed the first such extraction by using his thumb at the inferior limbus to drive the cataract out of the eye (1). In 1894, Dr. Eugene Kalt of Paris introduced the element of control by devising and using a capsule forceps (1). It is difficult to define the special set of circumstances that is needed before a bold new step in any operative procedure is introduced. Certainly one element must be the honest recognition by the inventor that the risk of complications associated with one of the steps is too high. This recognition must be coupled with a new technique that might improve the results. The new technique usually comes from some discovery made in a totally different branch of science or medicine. Such must have been the circumstances in 1867, when Henry Willard Williams of Boston (1) recognized the unacceptably high incidence of endophthalmitis connected with cataract surgery and realized that some sort of suture closure at the end of the operation might prevent the introduction of infection into the eye. One can only guess that his introduction of a sharp needle and fine suture for closure in cataract surgery must have sprung from some technological advance spawned by the American Civil

War. We think that Healon, too, falls into this paradigm of improvements in cataract surgery. Here, too, was the recognition that endothelial cell loss, particularly in a cornea with Fuchs' dystrophy, must be minimized. The idea of protectively coating tissues and prostheses had already been successfully demonstrated in the contact lens field where the use of wetting solutions allowed the lens to safely float over the cornea during a blink. In fact, Healon itself had come from the field of rheumatology where it had been shown to be both safe and effective as a lubricant if injected into the knee joints of horses suffering from traumatic arthritis (2).

This chapter will describe the steps of a typical intracapsular cataract extraction. However, interspersed throughout the chapter, an asterisk will introduce those sections containing the new steps in which Healon can be used to improve the results of the surgery. These are not idle claims, for it has already been demonstrated that Healon decreases endothelial cell loss in cataract surgery (3) as well as decreasing vitreous loss (4).

THE OPERATION
Preliminary Steps

This chapter will assume that the surgeon has premedicated the patient successfully, has prepared and draped the patient in a favored manner, and that a suitable form of anesthesia has already been applied.

Ocular Massage

Over 100 years ago, Pagenstecher (5) recognized that preoperative digital massage avoided certain operative complications. We now know (6,7) that intermittent pressure (e.g., 15 seconds on and 5 seconds off so as not to permanently occlude the retinal circulation) forces out free water from the vitreous body, thus decreasing its volume as well as forcing out aqueous. This effect can be further enhanced by using intravenous hyperosmotic agents such as mannitol or urea. Ocular massage also compresses the retrobulbar compartment of the orbit and produces hemostasis if a vessel was pierced during injection. This compression can be followed by the progressive endophthalmos associated with massage. Finally, the maneuver also helps distribute any injected anesthesia more quickly throughout the tissues.

Insertion of Speculum

Our only point here is to emphasize that no matter which speculum is used, care should be taken that it does not press on the eye. To ensure that no unnecessary pressure is introduced, a sterile tonometer should be placed on the eye before and after speculum introduction. Another method of checking for undue pressure is to sweep the fornices with a muscle hook to check for pressure contacts between globe and speculum.

Fixation Suture

The globe is rotated down and a 4-0 suture on a tapered noncutting needle is inserted underneath the tendon of the superior rectus muscle about 10 mm posterior to the limbus. Just prior to needle introduction, the tendon and overlying conjunctiva are grasped and tented upward with a large toothed forceps. To avoid the production of subconjunctival hematoma, we recommend careful visualization and avoidance of large conjunctival blood vessels as the toothed forceps is applied. If the suture is freely moveable after placement and tension on the suture draws the conjunctiva into pleats around the limbus, then the suture is too superficial and should be replaced.

Conjunctival Flap

The making of a conjunctival flap prior to penetration into the globe produces a number of benefits. Histologic evidence shows that the flap firmly adheres to both sides of the limbal wound by the first postoperative day (8) and that this conjunctival bridge is strengthened by newly laid down collagen during the healing period (9). Thus, the flap not only covers the potentially irritating suture knots, but offers structural support to the wound. Claims that the conjunctival flap prevents the rare catastrophic complications of endophthalmitis and epithelialization of the anterior chamber would require statistical proof using an enormous clinical series with controls. Such studies have yet to be conducted.

   To perform the popular limbus based flap, the conjunctiva and underlying Tenon's capsule are grasped with a fine toothed capsule (care taken to avoid obvious blood vessels) in the 12 o'clock position, some 4 mm posterior to the limbus. The tissue is tented upward and buttonholed with a blunt-tipped scissor posterior to the forceps. Blunt dissection with the scissors (using a gentle spreading motion) is performed until the limbus is reached. The flap is now continued, both temporally and nasally, around the limbus for about 150°. The flap is then reflected onto the cornea exposing the sclera. All small bleeders should be cauterized.

*Corneal Moistening

No matter how often the corneal surface is irrigated with a physiologic saline solution, during the operation the epithelium will slowly become hazy and irregular. Thus, toward the end of the surgery, details within the anterior chamber will be more difficult to see and a keratometric reflection, which is used by some surgeons to control suture tension, will be irregular and difficult to evaluate. By placing a drop of Healon on the cornea and smearing it evenly over the surface, the cornea will remain clear and lustrous. This maneuver may be repeated before the actual cataract removal to guarantee a clear, lustrous cornea for the entire procedure.

Limbal Incision

To ensure globe immobility without the risk of producing a conjunctival hematoma during the incision, the surgeon should gently pull up on the superior rectus suture with one hand while the assistant places a counter pressure with a muscle hook in the inferior cul-de-sac. Globe immobility may also be accomplished by firmly grasping the superior rectus with a

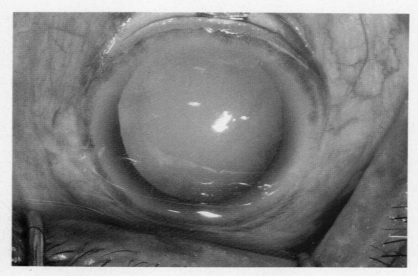

Figure 1. Fornix-based flap and appearance of a limbal groove.

large toothed forceps or by using a scleral pick. Once the globe is held steady, a blade with a half circle cutting tip is used to make a $^1/_2$ thickness groove around the superior limbus (at the junction of the blue and white zones) for about 150°. The groove serves three purposes. It allows the surgeon to insert accurately placed sutures prior to globe penetration (preplaced sutures), if this is the surgeon's preference. It acts as a guide for the scissors that will be used to complete the incision. Finally, it obviates the need to press the point of the razor blade knife forcefully through the entire limbal thickness to achieve penetration. At this juncture in the operation, a razor blade point is used to gently penetrate the floor of the groove and produce about a 3-mm entrance into the anterior chamber (Fig. 1).

*Protection of Iris and Lens

A fine cannula is mounted on the Healon syringe, and a small amount of Healon is instilled through the small limbal opening into the anterior chamber in order to push the superior iris and lens posteriorly. This maneuver will keep these structures away from the scissor blades, avoiding inadvertent punctures and tears.

The blades of the limbal scissors are then inserted into the wound and angled so as to give the wound the desired bevel. The completed incision should be between 120° to 180° in circumference (Fig. 2).

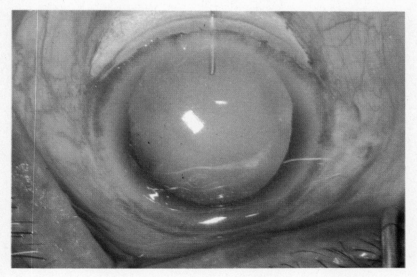

Figure 2. Appearance of Healon pushing iris and lens back.

Corneal Incision

There are a growing number of ophthalmic surgeons (10,11) who now advocate a clear corneal incision for the cataract operation. They feel that dispensing with the conjunctival flap eliminates annoying bleeding, gives better visualization of superior-anterior chamber structures, and allows more precise wound edge apposition. They further feel that a corneal section avoids trauma to the filtration structures, is easier to repair if a postoperative wound dehiscence occurs, and avoids trauma to a filtering bleb if one is present. However, a corneal section has certain disadvantages. It damages the endothelial cells adjacent to the incision, it heals more slowly (12), and it tends to produce higher levels of astigmatism until suture removal (13,14). Thus, with a corneal incision, the sutures usually have to be removed.

To make a corneal incision, the rounded knife is used to make a 180° groove in clear cornea, just central to the limbal vessels. A razor blade knife is then used to puncture the cornea.

*Protection of Iris and Lens with the Corneal Incision

A fine cannula is mounted on the Healon syringe and a small amount of Healon is instilled through the small corneal opening into the anterior chamber in order to protectively push the superior iris and lens pos-

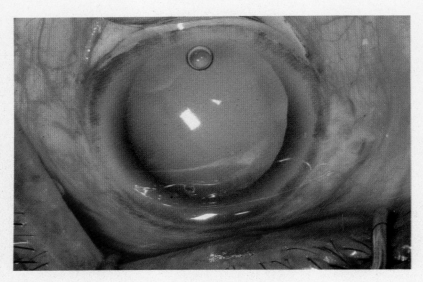

Figure 3. Anterior chamber deep with Healon in presence of large incision.

teriorly. This maneuver will keep these structures away from the scissor blade, avoiding inadvertent punctures and tears.

One blade of the corneal scissors is now inserted in the puncture site and angled to give the desired bevel and a 150°–180° incision is made. Dentate serrations in the wound can be avoided by not cutting down to the tips of the scissors (Fig. 3).

*Instrument Coating

To minimize instrument trauma to the corneal endothelium, the tips of all instruments placed into the anterior chamber should be lightly coated with Healon.

Peripheral Iridectomy

The tip of a fine, nontoothed forceps is gently slid past the incision, allowed to grasp the iris periphery, and a small triangle of iris is pulled out of the wound. Fine scissors are used to cut off the top of the iris triangle just below the forceps. The excised iris should then be spread out on the drape and the presence of pigment epithelium verified. Lack of such pigment implies that the iridectomy is only of partial thickness and must be completed.

Zonulolysis

Alpha-chymotrypsin, the enzyme introduced to ophthalmology by Professor Joaquin Barraquer (15) for zonulolysis, should be freshly prepared in a dilution of 1:5,000 to 1:10,000 just before the start of surgery. Since the enzyme is inactivated by blood, serum, epinephrine, and chloramphenicol (16), these substances must be irrigated from the chamber before instillation of the enzyme. 0.2 ml to 0.5 ml of the enzyme, placed in a syringe, should be introduced into the posterior chamber through the iridectomy or along the pupillary margin via an olive-tipped cannula. The drug brochure suggests that the enzyme be irrigated from the chamber two minutes after its introduction. However, some studies have shown that the enzyme is inactivated by aqueous humor (17,18) and, therefore, need not be irrigated out of the eye.

*Preparation of Olive-Tipped Cannula

Unfortunately, the olive-tipped cannula often scrapes off the pigment epithelium backing of the iris as it is advanced into the posterior chamber.

Such loss of pigment produces translucent patches of iris that will later splash scattered light onto the patient's retina, producing a dazzle glare. To prevent this rubbing off of pigment epithelium, the olive tip should be coated with Healon prior to insertion behind the iris.

Pause for Reevaluation

The next event will be the major event of the operation, that is, the extraction of the cataract. There are components of the extraction that can be traumatic to the corneal endothelium. For example, the cornea will have to be retracted to allow extraction. Such a maneuver both stretches the endothelial sheet at the crease and can dry the endothelium. As the cataract is drawn from the eye, the surface of the lens or the instrument that holds it may rub against the endothelial surface. Although most patients can afford the loss of some endothelial cells, about 10% of patients between 50 and 70 years of age go into the operating room with some degree of cornea guttata (19). The corneas of these patients may decompensate into an irreversible state of edema if significant numbers of cells are lost at surgery. To identify this group of vulnerable patients, preoperative endothelial cell counting can be performed if the surgeon suspects a problem. Preoperative corneal thickness measurements can also identify this group of high-risk patients. Studies suggest that any patient with a corneal thickness equal to or greater than 0.62 mm borders on corneal decompensation (20).

*Extra Corneal Endothelial Protection

In order to prevent endothelial loss, particularly in high-risk patients, enough Healon to coat the endothelial surface should be injected into the anterior chamber prior to the delivery of the cataract.

Intracapsular Cataract Extraction

At this point in the procedure, the respective roles of the surgeon and assistant are reviewed and silence is called for in the operating room. If a conjunctival flap has been made, the assistant will retract the cornea by grasping the flap with a fine toothed forceps. If a corneal section has been made, a 7-0 suture should have been placed at 12 o'clock on the corneal flap. The assistant should grasp both ends of the suture with a nontoothed forceps and gently retract the cornea. The assistant should also have a small bottle of physiologic salt solution, armed with an irrigating cannula, poised and ready to irrigate any tissue that inadvertently sticks to the cryoextractor. The surgeon now retracts the iris, thus en-

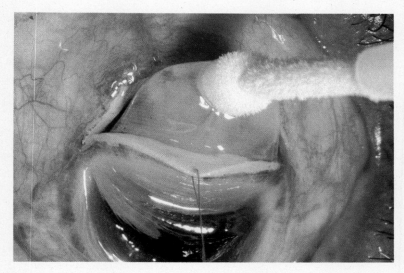

Figure 4. The cryoextraction of the cataract in an intracapsular fashion.

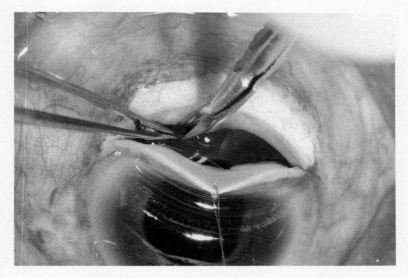

Figure 5. Production of a peripheral iridectomy.

larging the pupil, with either a cellulose sponge or an iris retractor. In patients who have been chronic miotic users, the pupil remains rigid and small. Thus, safe delivery of the cataract can only be accomplished with a full sector iridectomy. The tip of the cryoextractor, in the non-frozen state, is then plunged through the anterior chamber until it firmly engages the surface of the cataract midway between anterior pole and lens equator. At this point, the surgeon activates the freezing mechanism and waits for a solid ice ball connection to develop between lens and cryophake. Once a solid connection is achieved, a combination of rotary and rocking movements are used to slowly pull the lens out of the incision. If the lens refuses to yield and the lens capsule shows deep stretch creases, then the assistant must be ready to place a muscle hook or the cannula on the irrigating bottle on the inferior limbus at an angle of 45° and, under the surgeon's guidance, gently press the cataract out through the incision (Figs. 4 and 5).

*Erisiphake Extraction

In the event that an erisiphake is used, the back surface should be coated with Healon in order to prevent scraping of the endothelial surface during cataract delivery.

Wound Evaluation

At this stage in the operation, the wound edges should be evaluated. Is free vitreous present in the wound? Is the vitreous body bulging forward? Is the vitreous simply just below the cornea or is it pushing the wound open? Is the vitreous retracted so far posteriorly that the cornea is in a concave configuration? Is the iris in the wound?

If free vitreous is in the wound, then an anterior vitrectomy must be completed until almost no vitreous is in the anterior chamber and the cornea almost adopts a concave shape.

*Mildly Bulging Vitreous–Iris Diaphragm

If the vitreous–iris diaphragm takes on a convex configuration and lurks just below the cornea, Healon should be gently introduced into the anterior chamber. The Healon will act as a magic hand and push back the diaphragm in a stepwise fashion as it is slowly flushed across the chamber until the entire chamber deepens.

If the vitreous face has come far enough forward to force the wound edges apart, an anterior vitrectomy will have to be performed as if there were free vitreous in the wound (Figs. 6 and 7).

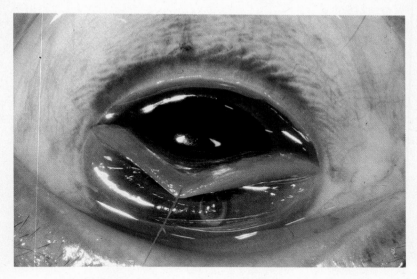

Figure 6. The appearance of a vitreous bulge.

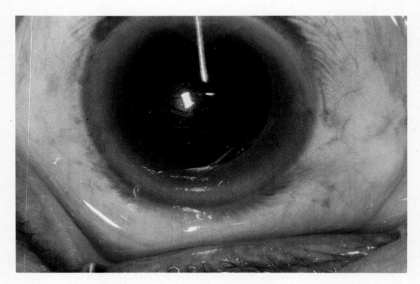

Figure 7. Introduction of the Healon to push back the vitreous-iris diaphragm.

*Iris Prolapse

If prolapsed iris is in the wound, placement of Healon into the anterior chamber will often push the body of the iris posteriorly, bringing the prolapsed portion of the iris with it. If this maneuver does not work, the prolapsed iris can be pushed back through the wound with a small spatula coated with Healon.

*Healon vs. Vitreous in the Wound

Just prior to wound closure, the wound edges must be inspected to make sure no vitreous is present. If Healon has been used, the surgeon may have difficulty differentiating Healon, which will not remain in the wound and cause problems (21), and vitreous. Certainly, both are transparent, both are sticky, and both are viscous. However, when the tip of a cellulose sponge is dipped into Healon and pulled up, the Healon will follow in a viscous string for 1–5 mm and then break. Because of its collagen matrix, vitreous will string out for a few centimeters before it snaps. If further confirmation is needed, a string of Healon is easily irrigated away with a jet of physiologic saline, whereas a string of vitreous is not (Figs. 8 and 9). Finally, as noted in Figure 8, a tug on a string of vitreous distorts the pupil. Tugging on a Healon string does not distort the pupil.

Wound Closure

There are many excellent suture materials that afford good closure. Fine silk remains the most popular because its pliability allows it to form such an easy knot. Fine nylon is useful because of its negligible tissue reactivity. Catgut, collagen, and polyglycolic acid sutures will dissolve in tissue and never need be removed. Fine stainless steel has great strength and stimulates the least amount of tissue reaction. On the other hand, silk can induce significant tissue reaction and may have to be removed. Nylon suture tends to compress a wound and may induce a significant astigmatism if not removed. The absorbable sutures lose most of their tensile strength long before a strong scar is formed and may allow microgaps in the wound. Such gaps occasionally lead to flat chambers or high astigmatism. Stainless steel sutures may also compress tissue and have to be removed. Thus, no suture material or method of suturing is perfect. At present, the use of 10-0 nylon is gaining in popularity at such a rapid rate, we decided to describe wound closure using this particular suture. By retaining its tensile strength over a long period of time, it can maintain a strong closure, even in the face of frequent use of local corticosteroids (which slow down wound healing). Each interrupted suture bite should

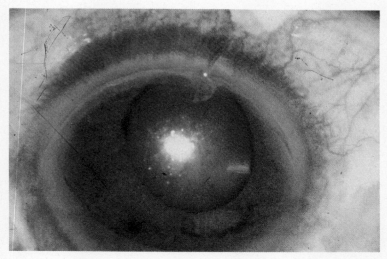

Figure 8. Strand of vitreous attached to cellulose sponge. Although vitreous and Healon are clear and viscous, they can be differentiated. The strand of vitreous is a few millimeters long and by pulling on it, the pupil will be noted to become distorted.

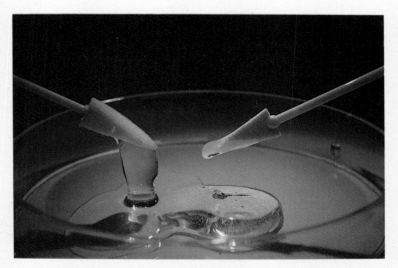

Figure 9. Photograph demonstrating difference between vitreous and Healon in vitro. A strand of vitreous attached to a cellulose sponge will stretch to a few millimeters. A strand of Healon attached to a similar sponge breaks after being extended about 1 millimeter or less.

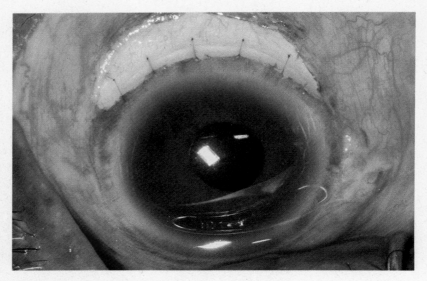

Figure 10. Wound closure with interrupted sutures (note the crystal clear cornea kept moist by Healon).

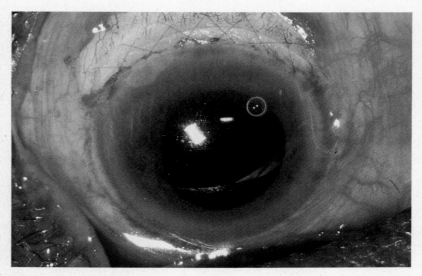

Figure 11. Wound closure with running sutures (note the crystal clear cornea kept moist by Healon).

be between 0.5 mm and 0.75 mm, should be about half thickness in depth, and should be placed a little less than one hour of the clock apart. The knot is made with an initial triple throw, followed by two single throws. The free ends are cut on the knot with a sharp razor blade. The knot of 10-0 nylon may then be pulled below the surface of the wound (Figs. 10 and 11).

*Wound Closure Under Keratometric Control

If the tension of each suture is determined by the reading of a surgical keratometer, a clear, nonconfusing reflection of the mires is very important. Air in the anterior chamber will produce an annoying second series of confusing reflections from the posterior corneal surface. However, Healon in the anterior chamber allows the cornea to maintain a domed shape and does not produce the secondary set of reflections. Healon in the anterior chamber can also tamponade a detachment of Descemet's membrane and restore corneal integrity.

Flap Closure

If a limbus-based flap was originally made, it should be closed with running 6-0 or 7-0 catgut suture. A fornix-based flap can be anchored nasally or temporally with interrupted fine catgut sutures or a cauterizing forceps.

Additional Measures

For complicated or traumatic operations, we recommend the use of subconjunctival corticosteroids (0.5–1.0 cc) and a subconjunctival antibiotic (0.5 cc). The superior rectus suture is then removed as well as the speculum. The eye is then gently closed and a double eye pad is taped tightly over the eye. A firm shield may also be placed over the pads for added protection.

REFERENCES

1. Duke Elder, S. *System of Ophthalmology.* St. Louis, C.V. Mosby, 1969, vol. 11, p. 248.
2. Miller, D. Healon. *Ann. Ophthalmol.* 13:781, 1981.
3. Pape, L.G., Balazs, E.A. Use of sodium hyaluronate (Healon) in human anterior segment surgery. *Ophthalmology* 87:699, 1980.

4. Choyce, P.D. Healon in anterior chamber implantation. *Am. Intraocular Implant Soc. J.* 7:138, 1981.

5. Pagenstecher, A. Über die Massage des Auges und deren Anwendung bei verschiedenen Augenkrankungen. *Centralbl. Prakt. Augenheilk* 2:281, 1878.

6. Hildreth, H.R. Digital ocular compression preceding cataract surgery. *Am. J. Ophthalmol.* 51:1237, 1961.

7. Francois, J., Gdal-On, M., Takeuchi, T., Victoria-Troncoso, V. Ocular hypertension and massage of the eyeball. *Ann. Ophthalmol.* 5:645, 1973.

8. Flaxel, J.T., Swan, K.C. Limbal wound healing after cataract extraction. *Arch. Ophthalmol.* 81:653, 1969.

9. Flaxel, J.T. Histology of cataract extraction. *Arch. Ophthalmol.* 83:436, 1970.

10. Pierse, D., Kersley, H.J. Microsurgery of cataract, vitreous and astigmatism. *Adv. Ophthalmol.* 33:173–200, 1976.

11. MacKensen, G. Microsurgical technique, in Kolder, H.E.J.W. (ed): *Proceedings of Paul Boeder International Symposium. Int. Ophthalmol. Clin.* 18:145, 1978.

12. Gassett, A.R., Dohlman, C.H. The tensile wound strength of corneal wounds. *Arch. Ophthalmol.* 79:595, 1968.

13. Jaffe, N.S. *Cataract Surgery and its Complications.* St. Louis, C.V. Mosby, 1981, p. 92.

14. Luntz, M.H., Livingston, D.G. Astigmatism in cataract surgery. *Br. J. Ophthalmol.* 61:360, 1977.

15. Barraquer, J. Enzymatic zonulolysis in lens extraction. *Arch. Ophthalmol.* 66:32, 1961.

16. Havener, W.H. *Ocular Pharmacology.* St. Louis, C.V. Mosby, 1970, p. 27.

17. Bedrossian, R.H., Weimar, V. Inhibitory effect of aqueous humor on alpha-chymotrypsin. *Trans. Am. Acad. Ophthalmol. and Otolaryngol.* 67:822, 1963.

18. Scheie, H., Yanoff, M., Tsou, K.C. Inhibition of alpha-chymotrypsin by aqueous humor. *Arch. Ophthalmol.* 73:399, 1965.

19. Kaufman, H.E., Capella, J.K., Robbins, J.E. The human corneal endothelium. *Am. J. Ophthalmol.* 61:635, 1966.

20. Miller, D., Dohlman, C.H. Effect of cataract surgery on the cornea. *Trans. Am. Acad. Ophthalmol. and Otolaryngol.* 74:300, 1970.

21. Arzeno, G., Miller, D. Effect of Na-hyaluranate on corneal wound healing. *Arch. Ophthalmol.* 100:152, 1982.

3

Extracapsular Cataract Extraction with Healon Using a Corneal Incision

Robert Stegmann

David Miller

Introduction

The logic of cataract fragmentation and aspiration through a small incision has attracted the ophthalmologist since Graeco-Roman times (1). However, the popularity of the procedure seems to have followed an enormous sine curve through history. Just when its popularity would wane, a new modification would be introduced and popularity would rise. Thus, when Teale (2) introduced mouth suction for more precise control, many London ophthalmologists adopted the technique. After a decline, an upsurge of interest followed Fuchs' (3) introduction of a double cannula so that simultaneous irrigation and aspiration could take place in almost a pressureless system. Scheie (4) repopularized the technique by providing maintenance of the anterior chamber with tight sutures around the cannula/syringe combination. The system was activated by a push-pull maneuver. Then Kelman (5) introduced high technology to the surgery by simultaneous fragmentation, irrigation, and suction under machine control. This method extended fragmentation and aspiration to many forms of adult cataracts that had previously resisted fragmentation. This last method requires exquisite control that must be maintained by frequent usage. At present, the popularity of the intraocular lens has again freshened our interest in extracapsular extraction.

45

The combination of an extracapsular extraction and lens implantation has been reported to produce a lower incidence of postoperative cystoid macular edema and lens dislocation when compared to lens implantation associated with an intracapsular extraction (6,7,8,9). Is there a way in which the ophthalmic surgeon with a modest surgical schedule can do the extracapsular extraction with a high level of safety? This chapter will describe a microsurgical technique that takes advantage of the viscoelastic sodium hyaluronate (Healon). This latter substance has proven very valuable in protecting corneal endothelium, deepening the anterior chamber, and pushing the vitreous face back during intraocular lens implantation (10,11). This chapter will describe the steps of extracapsular cataract extraction. Interspersed throughout the chapter will be the new steps, designated by an asterisk, in which Healon can be used to improve the results of the surgery.

The Study

The Healon method to be described was used on 20 patients and the results compared to 20 control patients who received a standard extracapsular extraction. The patients ranged from 16 to 50 years of age. Preoperative measurements included intraocular pressure and corneal thickness. Similar measurements were taken on the first postoperative day. Corneal endothelial cell counts were taken preoperatively and again one month postoperatively.

Of the 40 patients, every alternate patient received the concentric cannula irrigation–aspiration technique, as popularized by Scheie (4), using Ringer's lactate solution as the irrigant. The other 20 patients had irrigation–aspiration surgery using sodium hyaluronate to keep the chamber deep while the irrigation solution was used to aspirate the fragmented lens material.

Table 1. Effect of Extracapsular Cataract Extraction on Intraocular (IOP) Pressure

Number	Type of Surgery	Average IOP (mm Hg) ± S.D.
Preoperative		
20	Healon and aspiration	14.5 mm Hg ± 3.6
20	Ringer's and aspiration	15.0 mm Hg ± 2.1
Postoperative		
20	Healon and aspiration	13.25 mm Hg ± 3.7
20	Ringer's and aspiration	15.8 mm Hg ± 3.7

Table 2. Effect of Extracapsular Cataract Extraction on Corneal Thickness

Number	Type of Surgery	Average Corneal Thickness mm ± S.D.
Preoperative		
20	Healon and aspiration	0.51 mm ± .017
20	Ringer's and aspiration	0.52 mm ± .015
Postoperative		
20	Healon and aspiration	0.54 mm ± .016
20	Ringer's and aspiration	0.59 mm ± .017

The Results

Table 1 shows the pre- and postoperative intraocular pressure in both the control and Healon groups. No significant difference can be seen between the groups.

Table 2 shows the pre- and postoperative corneal thickness measurements in both groups. The postoperative corneal thicknesses in the control group were statistically thicker than the Healon group.

Table 3 compares the percentage of endothelial cells lost four weeks after surgery in each group. The increased cell loss in the control group is significantly greater than in the Healon group.

In determining the complication rate of a surgical procedure, one refers to articles written by very experienced surgeons describing large series of patients. We submit that such papers merely provide the lower limit of the complication rate. The average ophthalmic surgeon in the United States will do 50 cataract operations a year. Except for some very talented people, such surgeons will probably average a higher complication rate for a technically difficult operation like extracapsular cataract extraction. Thus, the average surgeon is more apt to traumatize corneal endothelium by prolonged irrigation or inadvertent instrument touch.

Table 3. Endothelial Cell Loss after Extracapsular Cataract Extraction

	Healon		Saline
No. cases	20		20
Mean	6.3%		13.9%
Standard deviation	3.3%		5.2%
Differences of mean		7.6%	
Significance of differences		0.01 level	

The same surgeon may also experience more posterior capsule rupture as well as posterior hyaloid rupture because of inadvertent high irrigation pressure. The use of the viscoelastic sodium hyaluronate maintains a deep anterior chamber, protectively coats corneal endothelium, and helps to dampen overenthusiastic irrigation pressure, thus preventing capsule rupture.

EXTRACAPSULAR CATARACT EXTRACTION WITH HEALON

Preliminary Steps

A successful extracapsular extraction is heavily dependent on maximal mydriasis. Thus, two hours before surgery, the eye to be operated on receives one drop of 1% Mydriacyl and one drop of 2.5% or 10% phenylephrine every 15 minutes. This sequence is repeated six times.

The most effective anesthesia is left to the surgeon's discretion, as well as the use of intravenous osmotic agents.

After the preparation and draping of the patient in the surgeon's accustomed manner, ocular massage is used for five minutes to help shrink the vitreous body.

A favored lid speculum is placed in the eye. A muscle hook may be used to sweep the fornices to see that there are no pressure contacts between globe and speculum.

A superior rectus stay suture is then inserted to help immobilize the eye. To avoid a subconjunctival hematoma, careful visualization through the operating microscope or a loupe is used to guarantee that the teeth of the forceps avoid sizable blood vessels as the tendon of the superior rectus is grasped.

*Corneal Moistening

Since Healon resists evaporation about 4 times more effectively than physiologic salt solution, it is very effective at keeping the corneal surface moist and clear. Thus, a drop of Healon is placed on the corneal apex and gently rubbed over the entire surface. This should keep the cornea clear and lustrous for 15 to 20 minutes.

Corneal Incision

Using a rounded knife, a 150°–180° groove is made on the corneal side of the limbus, central to limbus vessels. A razor blade incision of 3 mm is made at 12 o'clock along the floor of the groove. The incision is extended to 165° with corneal scissors.

*Maintenance of a Deep Chamber

A small amount of aqueous is allowed to escape from the anterior chamber. Then sodium hyaluronate is introduced through a small cannula into the anterior chamber before completion of the section, thus pushing iris and lens away from the tips of the scissors. This maneuver will maintain a deep chamber, although a large incision is present (Figs. 1 and 2).

Peripheral Iridectomy

The tip of a fine, nontoothed forceps is now gently slid past the incision and allowed to grasp the iris periphery. A small triangle of iris is pulled from the wound and cut. The excised iris should be spread over the drape and the presence of pigment verified. If no pigment is present, the iridectomy is not complete.

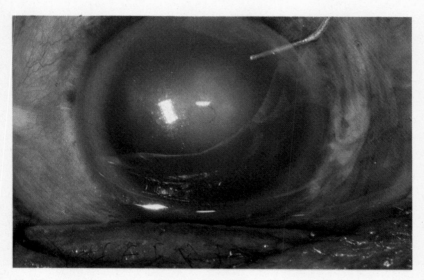

Figure 1. Introduction of Healon into the anterior chamber to push iris back.

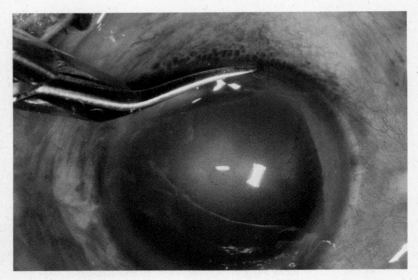

Figure 2. Corneal scissors making clear corneal section (note how iris is kept back).

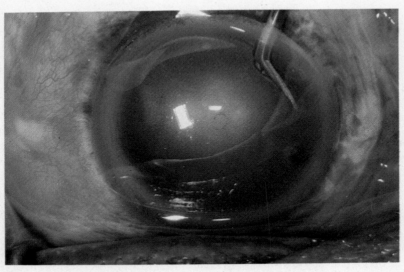

(a)

Figure 3. The making of a capsulotomy using fine scissors (chamber filled with Healon). (*a*) Superior nasal position; (*b*) superior temporal position; (*c*) completed anterior capsulectomy.

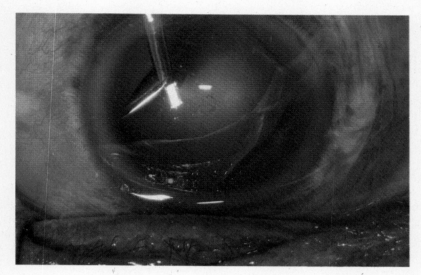

(b)

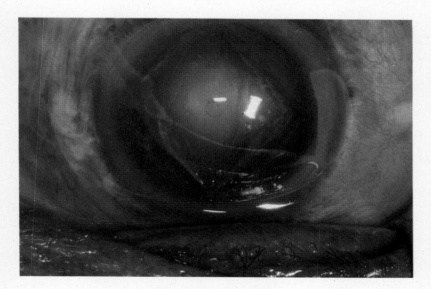

(c)

Figure 3. (Continued)

*Extracapsular Extraction

A sharp cystotome or bent 27-gauge needle is introduced into the incision, and an anterior capsulotomy is performed by making 16 radial cuts all around the lens, just central to the wide pupillary opening. An anterior capsulotomy may also be performed with fine scissors (Fig. 3). The capsule fragment is then grasped and removed with a fine forceps. Gentle pressure at 6 o'clock is now used to prolapse the nucleus and push it out through the incision. This maneuver may be facilitated by placing a lens loop under the nucleus and lifting it out (Fig. 4).

Irrigation–Aspiration

A modern irrigation–aspiration 19-gauge cannula with a 3.0 mm aspiration side port is attached to a 10-cc syringe filled with balanced salt solution and is used to remove the remaining cortex in a push-pull fashion. The small port allows selective aspiration of cortical remnants and the viscous Healon, minimizing chamber collapse. If the chamber starts to shallow, Healon is pumped in to restore its depth.

By irrigating Healon behind the anterior capsule and floating it forward, peripheral cortical remnants can easily be visualized and then removed. For example, remaining cortex at 12 o'clock is removed by reinserting the Healon-filled syringe attached to the 30-gauge cannula and instilling a small amount through the iridectomy, which separates iris from intact posterior capsule. Then the 19-gauge aspirating cannula is reintroduced through the iridectomy under the anterior capsule and the cortical remnants removed.

The lens cortex mixes easily with the sodium hyaluronate almost drawing the pieces of lens into the viscoelastic matrix. Healon may have to be introduced one to four times to maintain the chamber.

As a last step, a sandblasted flat cannula is used to gently and meticulously scrape off the final material from the posterior capsule.

The viscous quality of Healon maintains the anterior chamber throughout the procedure, thus helping to keep the cannula or any hard nuclear material from touching the corneal endothelium (Figs. 5, 6, 7, and 8).

*Healon vs. Vitreous in the Wound

In the event that the posterior capsule is punctured and vitreous escapes from the wound, how can the surgeon differentiate between the clear and viscous Healon and the clear and viscous vitreous? If the tip of a cellulose sponge is dipped into Healon and pulled up, the Healon will

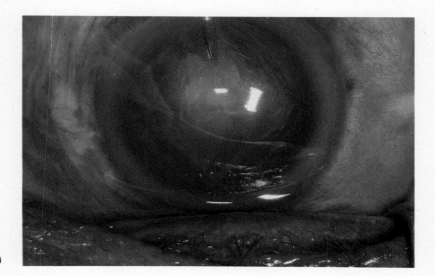

(a)

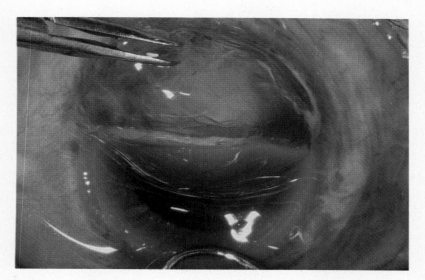

(b)

Figure 4. The nucleus expression using a lens loop. (a) Initial maneuver in which anterior capsule is removed; (b) nucleus partially expressed.

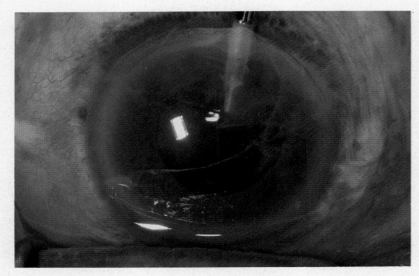

Figure 5. Use of the McIntyre cannula for aspirating cortical material activated by hand-held syringe.

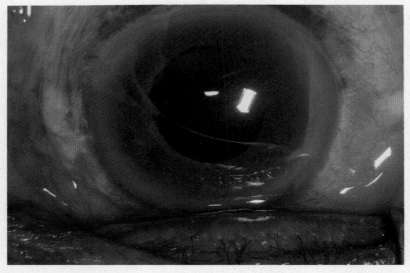

Figure 6. Maintenance of anterior chamber with Healon throughout procedure.

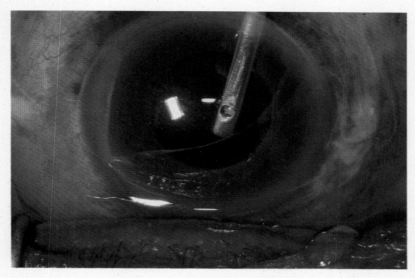

Figure 7. Gentle cleaning of posterior capsule under Healon blanket.

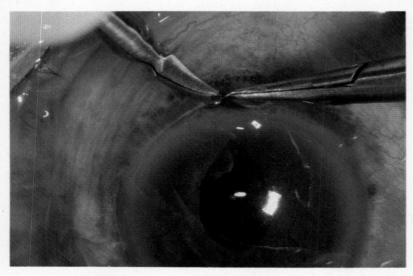

Figure 8. Making of a peripheral iridectomy.

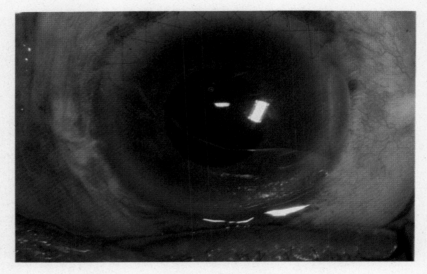

Figure 9. Wound closure with running suture.

follow in a thick string for 1–5 mm and then break. Because of its collagen matrix, vitreous will string out for a few centimeters before it snaps. If further confirmation is needed, a string of Healon is easily irrigated away with a jet of physiologic saline, while vitreous is not. Finally, pulling on a string of vitreous will usually distort the pupil, whereas pulling on a string of Healon will not distort the pupil.

Wound Closure

Once the anterior chamber is clean of lens material, the remaining Healon is left in the eye and the incision closed with interrupted 9 or 10-0 nylon sutures. Each suture is knotted with a triple throw followed by two single throws. The ends are cut right on the knot with a razor blade. The knot is then pulled into the stroma with a nontoothed forceps (Fig. 9).

REFERENCES

1. Ziegler, S.L. History of discission of the lens with the technique of complete discission by the V-shaped method. *Trans. Ophthalmol. Soc. U.K.* 45:154, 1925.
2. Teale, T.P. On extraction of soft cataracts by suction. *Lancet* 2:348, 1864.

3. Fuchs, J. Die zweiwegespritze ein neuartiges instrument zur absaugung weicher stare. *Klin. Monatsbl. Augenheilkd.* 121:592, 1952.

4. Scheie, H.G. Aspiration of congenital or soft cataracts: A new technique. *Am. J. Ophthalmol.* 50:1048, 1960.

5. Kelman, C.D. Phaco-emulsification and aspiration: A new technique of cataract removal. A preliminary report. *Am. J. Ophthalmol.* 64:23, 1967.

6. Binkhorst, C.D. The iridocapsular (two loop) lens and the iris clip (four loop) lens in pseudophakia. *Trans. Am. Acad. Ophthalmol. and Otolaryngol.* 77:589, 1973.

7. Binkhorst, C.D., Kats, A., Tjan, T.T., et al. Intracapsular vs. extracapsular surgery. *Trans. Am. Acad. Ophthalmol. and Otolaryngol.* 83:120, 1976.

8. Jaffe, N.S. Results of intracapsular implant surgery, in *Symposium on Cataracts, Trans. New Orleans Acad. Ophth.* St. Louis, C.V. Mosby, 1979, p. 310.

9. Miller, D., Stegmann, R. Use of Na-hyaluronate in anterior segment surgery. *Am. Intraocular Implant Soc. J.* 6:13, 1980.

10. Miller, D., O'Connor, P., Williams, J. Use of Na-hyaluronate during intraocular lens implantation in rabbits. *Ophthalmic Surg.* 8:58, 1977.

11. Binder, P.S., Sternberg, H., Wickham, M.G., Worthern, D.W. Corneal endothelial damage associated with phacoemulsification. *Am. J. Ophthalmol.* 82:48, 1976.

12. Sugar, J., Mitchelson, J., Kraff, M. The effect of phacoemulsification on corneal endothelial density. *Arch. Ophthalmol.* 96:446, 1978.

4

Extracapsular Cataract Extraction by Phacoemulsification Using Healon

Bo Philipsson

Ake Holmberg

Introduction

After the popularization of cryoextraction by Krwawicz in 1961 (1), it was felt that the ultimate method of intracapsular cataract surgery had been developed. The results of cryoextraction have been very good in the hands of experienced surgeons, and, furthermore, this type of extraction has been relatively simple to learn.

In spite of the high success achieved with existing methods, the advantages of extracting the lens through a small incision to minimize wound closure problems and astigmatism led to the development of a new procedure. Kelman (2) was the first to succeed in making such a procedure possible, even for extraction of relatively hard senile cataracts.

The first commercial Cavitron/Kelman Phaco-Emulsifier and Aspirator System was introduced in 1970. Since then the method has created a great deal of discussion, albeit not all in favor of the method. There is no doubt, however, that the phacoemulsification procedure has shown the advantages of a small incision and has also lowered the rate of vitreous and retinal complications of cataract surgery by saving all or most of the posterior lens capsule.

In the hands of a highly skilled surgeon, phacoemulsification is as safe or even safer than conventional cataract surgery. For the novice, however, it is a difficult technique to learn. Previous surgical experience is of limited or little value. Almost every step of the procedure is new, and the margin for error and variation is small. In the early series of patients operated on with phacoemulsification, the rate of complications was reported as high (2–4). Temporary postoperative corneal edema was observed very frequently, and occasionally even permanent corneal edema was seen. With growing experience the complication rate decreased, but it seemed as if this technique, irrespective of surgical experience, caused more damage to the corneal endothelium than conventional surgery (5–8). In experimental studies (9–11) on cats and rabbits, it was shown that mechanical trauma was likely to be the most important factor in causing corneal damage. Maneuvering of instruments in the anterior chamber and manipulating the lens nucleus or fragments of the lens nucleus in the anterior chamber during emulsification involved a great risk of damaging the corneal endothelium. Irrigation–aspiration or ultrasound within the time limits used during the procedure seemed to be of minor importance in inducing corneal damage. By performing the emulsification of the lens nucleus in the posterior chamber the corneal damage could be reduced. Still, for the surgeon who is learning the technique, phacoemulsification may pose hazardous risks to the corneal endothelium.

To explore the use of Healon in cataract surgery without intraocular lens (IOL) implants, a prospective study was begun in early 1980 involving three different surgical techniques, where extracapsular cataract extraction by phacoemulsification in the anterior chamber was included. The study was doubleblind with age-matched patients as controls. In the control patients balanced salt solution (BSS) was used instead of Healon.

The results obtained so far have been summarized in Table 1. The

Table 1. Data from the Clinical Trial of Healon with Age-Matched Controls[a]

Treatment Group	CCT (% of Preop) 1 Day Postop	CECD (% of Preop) 40 Days Postop	IOP (Difference from Preop) 1 Day Postop
BSS	142 ± 7	63 ± 10	− 1.1 mm Hg ± 1.9
Healon	125 ± 8	82 ± 9	+ 2.9 mm Hg ± 3.9

[a]Postoperative mean values and the standard error of the mean are given for central corneal thickness (CCT), central endothelial cell density (CECD), and intraocular pressure (IOP).

study shows that phacoemulsification in the hands of beginners causes considerable damage to the cornea, resulting in significant postoperative corneal edema and a substantial loss of corneal endothelial cells.

The study also shows that Healon can reduce the damaging effect of the procedure to about the same level as conventional cataract surgery (12–15).

Increase of intraocular pressure (IOP) after the use of Healon in cataract surgery has been reported (16,17). We have also observed a rise in IOP on the first day postoperatively after use of Healon in a few patients, but in general Healon does not affect IOP. Injection of excessive amounts, however, might occasionally result in an increase of IOP. No other side effects of Healon, such as the prolonged postoperative in-flammatory reaction reported by Binkhorst (16), were observed.

This study and the use of Healon in a large number of our patients have given us some experience in the use of Healon in the phacoemul-sification procedure.

NORMAL PHACOEMULSIFICTATION PROCEDURE

The phacoemulsification procedure has been excellently described in detail by Kelman (18) and Emery and Little (19).

A brief summary of the main steps in the procedure without use of Healon will be given. At each step the possible usefulness of Healon will be described.

1. Incision. Generally a short 3-mm-wide corneoscleral incision is made either under a limbal- or fornix-based, small conjunctival flap. The incision is made in the gray line parallel to the plane of the iris.

Healon use: Healon is generally not needed at this stage.

2. Anterior capsulectomy. A cystotome (Fig. 1) is used to cut the anterior capsule. The cystotome is attached to a flask containing irrigating fluid, generally BSS. By setting the flask at about 65 cm above the level of the eye, the anterior chamber can be kept deep. If no capsule-fixed IOL is to be introduced, the capsule is cut as far out as possible. Generally, small cuts are performed to achieve a large and continuous capsulec-tomy. A wide pupil (about 8mm in diameter) is very important for all steps in the procedure.

For the beginner, however, it is not unusual for the depth of the anterior chamber to vary considerably, and sudden collapse of the anterior chamber occurs not infrequently. During any of these manipu-lations, the corneal endothelium can easily be damaged.

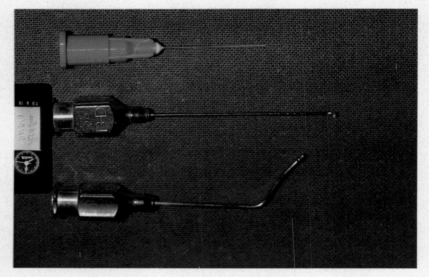

Figure 1. Instruments for capsulectomy and luxation of lens nucleus. Top: disposable needle (27-gauge) with a bent tip; middle: cystotome with irrigation; bottom: tire tool spatula with irrigation.

Healon use. Replacement of the aqueous humor with Healon has several advantages during the capsulectomy procedure: the anterior chamber can be kept deep, there are no fluctuations of the anterior chamber depth, nor is there risk of a sudden collapse of the anterior chamber. There is also no need for irrigation. All these facts contribute to minimize the risk of damaging the corneal endothelium with the instruments. Furthermore, Healon prevents the lens cortex from protuding into the anterior chamber, which makes the capsulectomy easier to perform. Finally, Healon (simply because of its viscosity) helps to keep the pupil well dilated. After the corneoscleral incision is made, the anterior chamber is filled with Healon (about 0.2 ml). It is important that the filling starts in the lower part of the anterior chamber, so that aqueous humor is pushed out through the incision and is totally replaced by Healon (Fig. 2). The anterior capsulectomy can now be performed without irrigation, and the pupil is often further dilated. The cuts are best performed with the bent tip of a disposable needle (27 gauge, Fig. 3). The needle is attached to the cystotome handpiece without the use of irrigation. Small and continuous cuts are done in the capsule at the edge of the widely dilated pupil.

   3. Prolapse of the lens nucleus into the anterior chamber. For the beginner, it is advisable to dislocate the nucleus into the anterior chamber. This

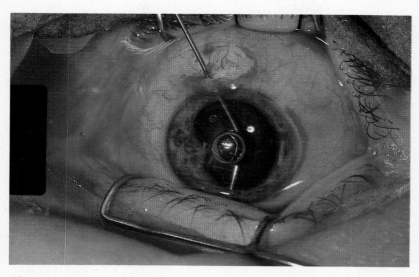

Figure 2. The aqueous humour is replaced by Healon before the capsulectomy. The filling starts in the lower part of the anterior chamber. A 27- to 30-gauge cannula is used. About 0.2 ml Healon is injected. The patient has a traumatic cataract with posterior synechia.

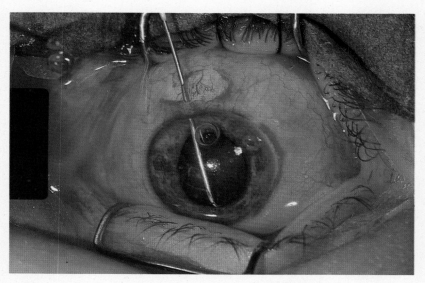

Figure 3. Anterior capsulectomy with the use of Healon. A thin disposable needle with bent tip is used without irrigation. Same patient as Figure 2.

can generally be performed by the capsulotome or with the help of a tire-tool spatula (Fig 1).

Healon use. Even during this step it is important that the anterior chamber stays deep and the pupil be well dilated. In addition, it is essential that the nucleus does not rub against the corneal endothelium. During this procedure, Healon has the same favorable effect as during the capsulectomy and, in addition, Healon acts as a protective layer between the endothelium and the nucleus. Usually there is no need to inject more Healon, since most of that injected for capsulectomy will remain in the anterior chamber. Healon can even be used to help dislocate the nucleus into the anterior chamber.

4. Phacoemulsification of the lens nucleus in the anterior chamber with the ultrasound tip. During emulsification great care must be taken not to touch the endothelium with the instrument tip, with the nucleus, or with pieces of the nucleus. The iris should, of course, not be touched, but a slight depigmentation resulting from iris touch is less dangerous than touching the corneal endothelium. In order to avoid damage to the cornea and the iris, it is important to keep the anterior chamber deep.

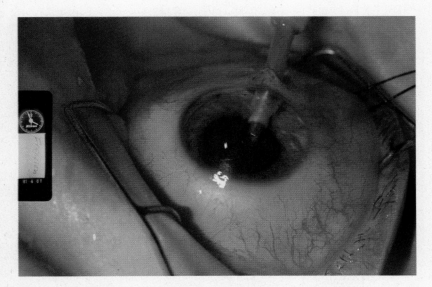

Figure 4. When introducing the ultrasound tip, the anterior chamber must be deep. Healon is of great value during this maneuver in protecting the endothelium.

Healon use. Most Healon injected during the capsulectomy remains in the anterior chamber and keeps it deep. It is most important to have a deep anterior chamber when the ultrasound tip is introduced into the incision, so as not to touch the endothelium (Fig. 4). Healon will probably be washed out from the anterior chamber by the irrigation–aspiration action of the phacoemulsifier. It is therefore questionable if Healon is of any help during emulsification. It is possible, however, that despite constant irrigation a thin layer of Healon sticks to the endothelium and gives some protection. In any case, Healon has no adverse effects during this stage. One way of reducing possible corneal damage is to perform the phacoemulsification in the posterior chamber. After the anterior capsulectomy, the nucleus is loosened but left in place. The emulsification is then performed in the posterior chamber.

5. *Aspiration of remaining cortical material* is performed with the irrigation–aspiration handpiece. This is an excellent instrument, and generally almost all cortical material can be aspirated (Fig. 5). This is a relatively safe procedure, but the amount of irrigating fluid should be limited to about 200 ml, including the irrigation during the phacoemulsification and capsulectomy procedure.

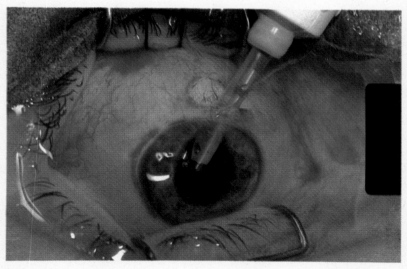

Figure 5. Aspiration of cortical remnants with the irrigation–aspiration instrument. Normally, Healon is not used during this procedure.

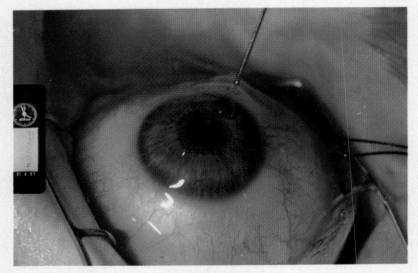

Figure 6. Repositioning of iris is easily performed with Healon.

Healon Use. Healon is not regularly injected during the normal irrigation–aspiration procedure.

6. *Closure of the incision* should be tight and can preferably be done with a 10-0 nylon suture placed as an X-suture.

Healon is of value in the following complications which may arise during the operation.

Break of posterior capsule. Vitreous loss. Vitrectomy. In conventional cataract surgery Healon is of considerable value in manipulating vitreous in the anterior chamber. For instance, a prolapsed vitreous can easily be pushed back with Healon. After a vitrectomy Healon prevents further prolapse of vitreous, and vitreous strands in the wound can also be removed more easily.

Iris prolapse. Repositioning a prolapsed iris is best made with Healon. No instruments should be used that may damage the iris. In fact, there is no need to introduce instruments into the anterior chamber. Healon also keeps the iris away from the wound; this facilitates suturing (Fig. 6).

Healon can be used to reform the anterior chamber. At the end of the operation the anterior chamber may be reformed with Healon. Care should be taken, however, not to inject too much Healon, more than 0.25 ml may cause a rise of IOP postoperatively. We find it is not necessary to wash out Healon at the end of an operation.

Conclusions

The main advantage gained in using Healon in all types of cataract surgery is in keeping the anterior chamber deep. This is especially important during phacoemulsification procedures, but Healon also has additional advantages such as reducing the amount of irrigation fluid needed and physically protecting the endothelium.

Phacoemulsification in the hands of a beginner induces a considerable amount of damage in the corneal endothelium. Our study shows that Healon, even during the phacoemulsification procedure, can act as an effective protective agent. Apart from this, we have found Healon especially useful during several phases of the procedure. For the novice Healon represents a kind of a safeguard, and it makes the surgeon more secure and relaxed and several of the maneuvers less critical.

The different phases of the phacoemulsification technique can, of course, be handled properly by a skilled surgeon without Healon. As mentioned earlier, however, the technique is difficult to learn, and a beginner will remain a beginner for a considerable period of time. For the novice Healon is definitely of great value, not only in facilitating several of the steps of the procedure, but also in acting as a protector of the corneal endothelium. In this way Healon may help popularize this new technique, which indeed has many advantages compared to conventional cataract surgery.

REFERENCES

1. Krwawicz, T. Intracapsular extraction of intumescent cataract by application of low temperature. *Br. J. Ophthalmol.* 45:279,1961.
2. Kelman, C.D. Phacoemulsification and aspiration. *Am. J. Ophthalmol.* 64:23, 1967.
3. Hiles, D.A., Hurite, F.G. Results of the first year's experience with phacoemulsification. *Am. J. Ophthalmol.* 75:473, 1973
4. Kelman, C.D. Phacoemulsification and aspiration. *Am. J. Ophthalmol.* 75:764, 1973.
5. Polack, F.M., Sugar, A. The phacoemulsification procedure: III. Corneal complication. *Invest. Ophthalmol. Vis. Sci.* 16:39, 1977.
6. Sugar, J., Mitchelson, J., Kraff, M. The effect of phacoemulsification on corneal endothelial cell density. *Arch. Ophthalmol.* 96:446, 1978.
7. Irvine, A.R., Kratz, R.P., O'Donnell, J.J. Endothelial damage with phacoemulsification and intraocular lens implantation. *Arch. Opthalmol.* 96:1023, 1978.
8. Abbot, R.L., Foster, R.K. Clinical specular microscopy and intraocular surgery. *Arch. Ophthalmol.* 97:1476, 1979.
9. McCarey, B.E., Polack, F.M., Marshall, W. The phacoemulsification procedure: I. The effect of intraocular irrigation solutions on the corneal endothelium. *Invest. Ophthalmol.* 15:449, 1976.

10. Polack, F.M., Sugar, A. The phacoemulsification procedure: II. Corneal endothelial damage. *Invest. Ophthalmol.* 15:458, 1976.

11. Binder, P.S., Sternberg, H., Wickman, M.G., Worthen, D.M. Corneal endothelial damage associated with phacoemusification. *Am. J. Ophthalmol.* 82:48, 1976.

12. Pape, L.G., Balazs, E.A. Final report on the use of Healon® in cataract viscosurgery. *Ophthalmology* 86:109, 1979.

13. Olsen, T. Corneal thickness and endothelial damage after intracapsular cataract extraction. *Acta Ophthalmol.* 58:424, 1980.

14. Pape, L.G., Balazs, E.A. The use of sodium hyaluronate (Healon®) in human anterior segment surgery. *Ophthalmology.* 87:699, 1980.

15. Holmberg, Å.S., Philipson, B.T. Na-hyaluronate in cataract surgery. To be published.

16. Binkhorst, C.D. Inflammation and intraocular pressure after the use of Healon® in intraocular lens surgery. *Am. Intraocular Implant Soc. J.* 6:340, 1980.

17. Pape, L.G. Intracapsular and extracapsular technique of lens implantation with Healon®. *Am. Intraocular Implant Soc. J.* 6:342, 1980.

18. Kelman, C.D. *Phacoemulsification and Aspiration: The Kelman Technique of Cataract Removal,* New York, Aesculapius, 1975.

19. Emery, J.M., Little, J.H. *Phacoemulsification and Aspiration of Cataracts.* St Louis, C.V. Mosby, 1979.

5

Anterior Chamber Lens Implantation Combined with the Use of Healon

G. William Lazenby

In American ophthalmology today, the intraocular lens is probably more discussed than any other subject. This is in spite of the furor over intracapsular versus extracapsular cataract surgery and the recent controversy over radial keratotomy. To verify the interest in intraocular lenses, one need only to observe the number of meetings and courses devoted to their use. Improvement in surgical techniques, instrumentation, and the lenses themselves have advanced the state of the art to such a point that it would appear that cataract surgery with intraocular lens implantation has no greater complication rate than cataract surgery alone.

The anterior chamber intraocular lens was first used by Strampelli, but it was D. P. Choyce who carefully improved the lenses through nine modifications. It was also Choyce who so thoroughly instructed many of us in his gracious home at Southend-on-Sea in England. Credit must also be given to Charles Kelman for modifications that allowed the anterior chamber intraocular lens to be inserted through a small incision making it amenable for use with phacoemulsification. The substitution of loops for solid polymethyl methylmethacrylate was in the author's opinion a great improvement in anterior chamber intraocular lens design. Not only was the lens made lighter, but the flexible loops greatly decreased the degree of tenderness felt by patients for months or years after the surgery. As a sequel to the introduction of loops on the lenses, we may soon have a lens that can be used equally well in the anterior or posterior chamber. This would indeed be the universal lens, since it would lend itself to use by intracapsular or extracapsular surgeons.

Since the use of intraocular lenses has become more or less general in the United States, probably no event has been more momentous than the discovery that Healon could be safely used in the anterior chamber. Because of its unique viscoelastic properties, Healon gave protection to the corneal endothelium which had not heretofore been possible with air or balanced salt solution. It has also been found that Healon makes anterior chamber intraocular lens placement much easier because of a dampening effect on the intraocular lens (1–7).

In a study we recently completed, 40 patients from our private practice participated. The study was undertaken primarily to determine the effect of Healon on endothelial cell loss in intracapsular cataract extraction with insertion of anterior chamber intraocular lens.

Preoperative examination included a general medical and ocular history together with a complete eye examination. Pachometry, keratometry, and endothelial cell counts were also carried out. All patients received 25 mg indomethacin with the evening meal the day before surgery. The following morning an intracapsular cataract extraction was performed. In the 19 eyes randomly chosen to receive hyaluronic acid, the anterior chamber was filled with Healon. In the 21 control eyes the anterior chamber was filled with balanced salt solution and air if necessary.

In all cases, the anterior chamber intraocular lens was then obliquely inserted from the temporal side. The distal end was carefully placed in the lower nasal angle followed by placement of the proximal end in the upper temporal angle. This was achieved by placing traction on the scleral lip to allow the proximal end to slide easily over the wound edge and onto the scleral spur. Thereafter, a peripheral iridectomy was performed and the wound was closed.

Table 1. Corneal Endothelial Cell Count[a]

	Preoperative	1 Month Postoperative	% Loss of Cells	
BSS (N = 21)	2397.6	2073.8	13.5	P<.01
Healon (N = 19)	2486.8	2244.7	9.7	P<.05

[a]In cells/mm². N.S. P .10

Table 2. Corneal Thickness[a]

	Preoperative	Postoperative	
BSS (N = 21)	0.69	0.69	N.S.
Healon (N = 19)	0.72	0.69	N.S.

[a]In mm. N.S. N.S.

Postoperative medication consisted of 1% atropine twice a day for approximately 60 days. Maxitrol suspension was given twice a day for approximately one week, and then replaced by fluorometholone (FML) suspension twice a day for usually 6 to 12 months. All subjects received 25 mg indomethacin three times a day for 20 days postoperatively. All subjects were then followed at 1–3 days, 1–2 weeks, 3–4 weeks, and 1–3 months postoperatively. Pachometry was performed at 1–2 weeks and postoperative corneal endothelial cell counts were performed at 1–3 months.

From Table 1 it can be seen that the endothelial cell loss in those patients receiving Healon was 9.7% while in the control subjects the cell loss was 13.5%. Although the cell loss with Healon was less, the difference was not statistically significant. From Table 2 it will be noted that corneal thickness was the same in Healon and control subjects. Although cell counts and corneal thickness did not appear to be measurably affected by Healon, it did contribute tremendously to the ease with which surgery was performed. As seen in Table 3, of the 19 patients treated with Healon, 16 were in the "easier" category and none were in the "more difficult" category. In contrast, of the 21 cases treated with balanced salt solution, only four fell into the "easier" category, while three were considered "more difficult." From these data, it can be seen that the majority of the surgery performed with Healon fell into the "easier" category.

Table 3. Surgeons Appraisal of Lens Implantation

	Easier	Average	More Difficult
BSS (N = 21)	4	14	3
Healon (N = 19)	16	3	—

$P<0.01$ $P<0.01$

DESCRIPTION OF PROCEDURE

It is recommended that each surgeon modify the cataract surgical procedure only to allow proper use of Healon. A description of the cataract extraction will not be included here for that reason.

*Reforming Anterior Chamber

After the cataract extraction the anterior chamber should be gently reformed by filling with Healon. It is important that the cannula be gradually advanced in the direction of flow as the chamber is filled. This is to avoid segmental deepening that could force vitreous out from a different area. This assumes even more importance in the presence of a bulging iridovitreal diaphragm, in which case one is trying gradually to force the vitreous and iris back far enough to allow safe lens insertion. One will immediately note that after the chamber has been adequately filled with Healon, the iris and vitreous will stay nicely posterior in spite of a possible bulging nature before insertion of Healon (Figs. 1, 2, and 3).

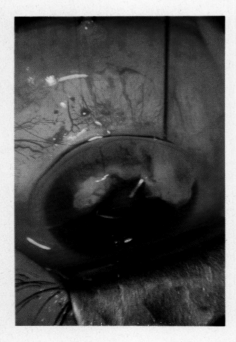

Figure 1. Retraction of cornea.

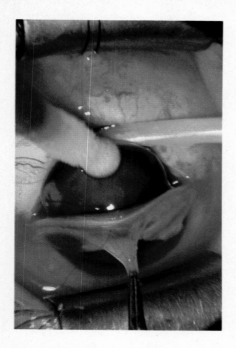

Figure 2. Cryoextraction of cataract.

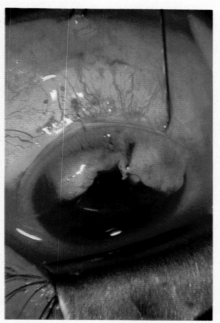

Figure 3. Appearance of iris-vitreal diaphragm.

Lens Insertion

Before inserting the anterior chamber intraocular lens, it is recommended that the anterior surface of the lens be covered with Healon.
This may be superfluous, but on the other hand it may give additional
protection to the corneal endothelium. The intraocular lens is then inserted from the upper temporal area. It should be gently thrust across
the anterior chamber and into the lower nasal angle with a single movement. At this point it will be noted that the intraocular lens is much
more stable than if balanced salt solution or air is used. The Healon has
a dampening effect that keeps the distal end of the lens under much
better control during the insertion. The distal end is also much more
easily maintained in proper position while the proximal end of the lens
is being maneuvered. The scleral lip of the wound is then retracted,
which will allow the proximal feet or loop of the intraocular lens to slide
easily over the wound edge and onto the scleral spur. The proper tests
should now be carried out to determine that the lens is in proper position
(Figs. 4, 5, and 6).

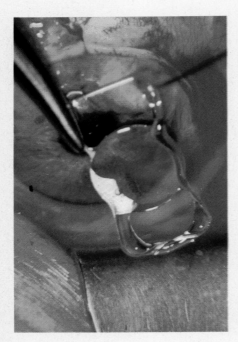

Figure 4. Coating the anterior chamber lens with Healon.

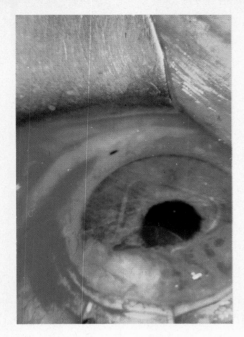

Figure 5. Sliding anterior chamber lens across iris plane.

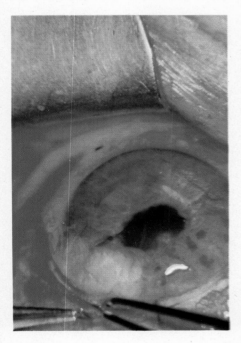

Figure 6. Tucking superior foot of anterior chamber lens under scleral shelf.

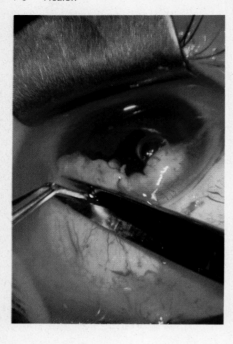

Figure 7. Making the iridectomy (after lens implantation).

Peripheral Iridectomy

The peripheral iridectomy should be performed after the intraocular lens is in place. If the iridectomy is performed before cataract extraction, there is greater risk of forcing vitreous through the iridectomy when filling the anterior chamber with Healon owing to the previously mentioned segmental deepening effect. Second, the iridectomy should be as far as possible away from the intraocular lens in case of slight rotational displacement in the postoperative period (Fig. 7).

*Final Anterior Chamber Irrigation

After it has been determined that the intraocular lens is in proper position and the iridectomy has been performed, the excess Healon should be gently washed from the anterior chamber with balanced salt solution to avoid elevated intraocular pressure in the postoperative period. Only enough Healon should be used to keep the anterior chamber deep enough for safe insertion.

CONCLUSION

It is probably safe to state that the effect of Healon will be to make the cataract operation with insertion of anterior chamber intraocular lens much easier to perform. This should make the surgeon feel more comfortable and in better control. The surgeon can now feel much more confident when faced with a cataract extraction combined with anterior chamber intraocular lens insertion.

REFERENCES

1. Balazs, E.A., Hultsch, E. Replacement of the vitreous with hyaluronic acid collagen and other polymers, in Irvine, O'Malley (eds): *Advances in Vitreous Surgery*. Springfield, II., Charles C Thomas, 1976, pp. 601–623.
2. Pape, L.G., Balazs, E.A. The use of sodium hyaluronate (Healon®) in human anterior segment surgery. *Ophthalmology* 87:699–705, 1980.
3. Balazs, E.A., Freeman, M.I., Kloti, R., et al. Hyaluronic acid and replacement of vitreous and aqueous humor. *Mod. Probl. Ophthalmol.* pp. 3–21, 1972.
4. Binkhorst, C.D. Inflammation and intraocular pressure after the use of Healon® in intraocular lens surgery. *Am. Intraocular Implant Soc. J.* 6:340–341, 1980.
5. Miller D., Stegmann, R. Use of Na-hyaluronate in anterior segment eye surgery. *Am. Intraocular Implant Soc. J.* 6:13–15, 1980.
6. Lazenby, G.W., Broocker, G. The use of sodium hyaluronate (Healon®) in intracapsular cataract extraction with insertion of anterior chamber intraocular lenses. Accepted for publication.
7. Pape, L.G. Intracapsular and extracapsular technique of lens implantation with Healon®. *Am. Intraocular Implant Soc. J.* 6:342–343, 1980.

6

Use of Healon in the Implantation of the Pupillary Plane Lens

Robert Stegmann

David Miller

Introduction

The first controlled study that demonstrated the advantages of Healon in intraocular lens implantation was performed using the Binkhorst 4-loop pupillary plane lens. Because the study provided such convincing proof of the usefulness of Healon, other ophthalmic surgeons were enlisted as investigators, and new uses for Healon were developed and confirmed at an amazing pace. To give the reader that sense of excitement that sparked the early investigators, it might be useful to review the conditions of that first study in some detail.

Twenty patients with severe bilateral mature cataracts, who requested bilateral intraocular implants, were selected for the study. The risks and benefits of being involved in the study were carefully explained and accepted by all 20 patients. Appropriate spacing between each operation was agreed upon with each individual patient. The surgery was all performed by one surgeon, using general anesthesia. The cataract extraction in all 40 eyes was of the intracapsular type, and the intraocular lens was always of the dry packaged Binkhorst iris clip variety. In a randomly determined fashion, one eye of each patient received an intraocular lens after the anterior chamber had been filled with sodium hyaluronate. The other eye received an intraocular lens using the conventional method of chamber maintenance, that is, saline and an air bubble.

Preoperative measurements in each eye included endothelial cell counts, visual acuity, corneal thickness (Haag Streit Pachometer), intraocular pressure (Applanation tonometer), and the state of the anterior chamber. Similar tests were recorded at postoperative days 1, 3, 7, 14, and 28. At the end of the postoperative month, central corneal endothelial cell counts (Heyer Schulte Endothelial Camera) were then repeated on each eye.

Postoperatively, all eyes of all patients received local steroid drops (q6h betamethasone) and local antibiotic drops (q6h Neosporin) for one month.

The average preoperative endothelial cell counts for each eye of the same individual were essentially the same (2810 cells/mm^2 vs. 2780 cells/mm^2).

At the end of one month, the average cell count for the group of eyes in which sodium hyaluronate was used was 2340 cells/mm^2 vs. 1250 cells/mm^2 for the control group. Thus, there was an average cell loss of 17% in the test eyes vs. a 54% cell loss in the control group of eyes. Using the Wilcoxon test, the difference in cell counts between both groups was statistically significant at the .01% level (see Table 1).

The corneal thickness for each group of eyes was statistically equal preoperatively at the .01 level, using the Wilcoxon test.

Refer to Table 2 for the actual differences between the two groups throughout the postoperative period. Note, however, that the control group of eyes were statistically thicker at the .01 level at every stage during the one month postoperative period.

The average corrected visual acuity was significantly better in the sodium hyaluronate treated eye throughout the one month postoperative period (see Table 3). For example, at postoperative day 1, the eyes treated with sodium hyaluronate averaged a corrected visual acuity of 20/160 vs. 20/1020 in the control group. At 7 days postoperative, the eyes treated with sodium hyaluronate averaged a corrected acuity of 20/60 vs. 20/120 in the control group.

Table 4 gives an account of the mean intraocular pressure for each group of eyes during the pre- and postoperative period. Note that the differences between the two groups was never significant.

Table 5 is a general summary of the entire study.

In both groups, a comparable mild anterior uveitis disappeared at the end of one week. Undoubtedly, the use of local steroids in both groups helped abate the uveitis by the first postoperative week. It should also be noted that cells in the anterior chamber appear frozen in place for the first two to three postoperative days because of the presence of Healon.

No synechiae developed between intraocular lens and iris in any of the 40 eyes.

Table 1. Corneal Endothelial Cell Count (per mm^2) After IOL
Implantation in Both Eyes of 20 Patients

Patient Number	*Healon*			*Saline*		
	Preop	*Postop*	*% Diff*	*Preop*	*Postop*	*% Diff*
1	2500	2200	12	2500	1200	52
2	3000	2500	17	2700	750	72
3	2700	2200	19	2700	750	72
4	3000	1500	50	3000	1500	50
5	3200	2500	22	3000	750	75
6	2500	2500	0	3000	2000	33
7	3000	2500	17	3000	750	75
8	2700	2500	7	3000	1000	67
9	3000	2700	10	3000	1000	67
10	2700	2200	19	2700	1700	37
11	3000	2200	27	3000	2000	33
12	2700	2000	26	2700	2000	19
13	2200	2200	0	2200	1000	55
14	3000	2500	17	3000	2500	17
15	2700	2200	19	2200	750	66
16	3200	2500	22	3200	1000	69
17	2500	2200	17	2200	1200	45
18	2700	2500	7	2500	1000	60
19	3200	3000	6	3200	1500	53
20	2500	2200	12	2500	750	70
Mean	2800	2300	18	2800	1300	54
±	300	300		300	500	

Significances		
Two Groups Compared (d.f. 19)	t	p
Healon preop–saline preop	0.75	NS
Healon preop–Healon postop	6.00	<0.001
Saline preop–saline postop	11.99	<0.001
Saline postop–Healon postop	7.11	<0.001

Only one dislocation occurred during the one month postoperative
period, and it was in an eye treated with sodium hyaluronate.
This event was not statistically significant.
Only one postoperative hyphema occurred (which resolved spontaneously) in a control eye. This event was not statistically significant. The

Table 2. Average Corneal Thickness (mm) After IOL Implantation in 20 Patients

	Preoperative	Postoperative				
		Day 1	Day 3	Week 1	Week 2	1 Month
Sodium hyaluronate	0.50	0.56	0.54	0.53	0.53	0.52
Saline	0.50	0.68	0.63	0.59	0.57	0.55
Significance	NS[a]	<0.01	<0.01	<0.01	<0.01	<0.01

[a]NS = Not significant

Table 3. Average Corrected Visual Acuity (Snellen) After IOL Implantation in 20 Patients

	Postoperative				
	Day 1	Day 3	Week 1	Week 2	1 Month
Sodium hyaluronate	20/160	20/80	20/60	20/50	20/40[a]
Saline	20/1020	20/410	20/120	20/80	20/30
Significance	<0.01	<0.01	<0.01	<0.01	NS

[a]This mean value is high because one eye in sodium hyaluronate group had preoperative senile macular degeneration (20/200) that could be diagnosed only after cataract surgery.

Table 4. Average Intraocular Pressure (mm Hg) After IOL Implantation in 20 Patients

	Preoperative	Postoperative				
		Day 1	Day 3	Week 1	Week 2	1 Month
Sodium hyaluronate	12 ± 0.4	9 ± 0.6	9 ± 0.5	10 ± 0.6	13 ± 0.6	13 ± 0.4
Saline	13 ± 0.4	8 ± 0.7	9 ± 0.6	12 ± 0.8	12 ± 0.9	13 ± 0.6
Significance	NS	NS	NS	NS	NS	NS

Table 5. Summary Data on IOP and Corneal Measurements Carried Out Before and After IOL Implantation in Both Eyes of 20 Patients

	IOP		Corneal Thickness		Visual Acuity (Corr)	Endothelial Cell Preop	Endothelial Count Postop[a]
	Preop	Postop[a]	Preop	Postop[a]			
Sodium hyaluronate	12 ±0.5	11 ±0.3	0.50 ±0.02	0.54 ±0.02	20/80	2800 ± 300	2300 ± 300
Saline	13 ±0.4	11 ±0.3	0.50 ±0.02	0.60 ±0.04	20/600	2800 ± 320	1300 ± 530
Significance	NS	NS	NS	<0.01		NS	<0.01

[a]Average of all postoperative measurements (1 day; 3 days, 1 week, 2 weeks, 1 month)

resorption of blood in the anterior chamber may be slightly delayed in the presence of Healon.

Two instances (one from each group) of postoperative choroidal detachment occurred leading to transient shallow chamber. These resolved in about four days.

The results clearly show that use of sodium hyaluronate produces endothelial cell loss (17%) comparable to routine cataract extraction without intraocular lens implantation as noted in the literature review (1). The endothelial cell loss found in our control eyes (54%) is also similar to that found in the literature review (1).

Most of the cataracts removed in this study were of the mature or hypermature variety. After cataract removal, the anterior vitreous face was noted to bulge forward in a high percentage of the cases. When sodium hyaluronate was instilled into the anterior chamber, it would push both iris and vitreous face back, thus deepening the chamber and making lens implantation easier technically. This added effect of chamber deepening with an open incision is a second benefit to the surgeon.

The study also showed that sodium hyaluronate did not induce a significant uveitis. Interestingly, at the end of the month less pigment dusting was noted on the anterior surface of the intraocular lens in those eyes in which sodium hyaluronate had been used. Thus, Healon may also have a mild anti-inflammatory effect.

THE PUPILLARY PLANE LENS

Introduction of a lens that depends upon the iris for support took place after the introduction of the posterior chamber lens and the anterior chamber lens. In the 1950s, E. Epstein of South Africa and C. D. Binkhorst of the Netherlands both introduced iris-fixated lenses of different designs. Epstein's maltese cross design is almost woven into the iris, while Binkhorst's iris clip design floats in aqueous but may strike the iris surface during eye movement (2). The Binkhorst lens was one of the first lenses introduced into the United States and was the subject of very extensive clinical evaluation. Jaffe (2) reported that about 90% of patients receiving this lens achieved a corrected visual acuity of 20/40 or better. The major causes of postoperative acuity of less than 20/40 were cystoid macular edema, corneal edema, and the presence of secondary pupillary membranes. It should also be noted that about 3% of Jaffe's series sustained a dislocation of the implant. All of these lenses were subsequently restored to the proper position.

The technique for implantation of the iris clip lens will now be described. Interspersed throughout the description of the technique will be headings introduced by an asterisk. These sections describe how the use of Healon will improve the results of the surgery.

IMPLANTATION OF THE PUPILLARY PLANE LENS USING HEALON

Preliminary Considerations

We will assume that the surgeon has moved smoothly through the operation and has just performed the intracapsular cataract extraction. Preoperative medication should have included six applications of 1% Mydriacyl and six applications of 10% phenylephrine, 15 minutes apart, to yield maximal mydriasis.

*Lens Implantation

A small mound of Healon is placed on the superior conjunctiva, and the intraocular lens is nestled within the mound. This coats the lens and keeps the lens in plain view of the surgeon. The anterior chamber is now filled with Healon. The filling should be gradual with the cannula slowly injecting the material as it advances from the superior limbus to the inferior limbus. As the Healon is injected, the vitreous–iris diaphragm is slowly pushed back across the entire chamber. The implant held within the mound of Healon is now grasped with a straight toothless tying forceps. The forceps should engage the body of the lens and the superior/anterior loop. The assistant now lifts the cornea high enough to allow introduction of the implant into the eye. The surgeon holds the lens at about a 45° angle with the iris plane and plunges the lens into the anterior chamber. His initial objective is to engage the inferior iris with the inferior loops. Once the inferior pupil is properly engaged, the lens is pushed gently toward the inferior limbus. The pupil is noted to elongate. This maneuver is continued until the superior/posterior loop just slips behind the superior pupil. It should be emphasized that the pupillary margin must not be stretched too strenuously during lens insertion. Vigorous stretching of the iris against a loop can lead to pressure damage of the pupillary sphincter (3). A damaged sphincter can lead to a poorly constricting pupil and a higher incidence of lens dislocation (4). The forceps is now slowly withdrawn from the wound. The surgeon

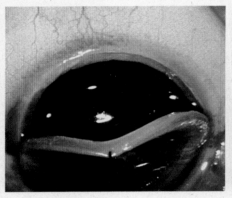

Figure 1. Bulging hyaloid face.

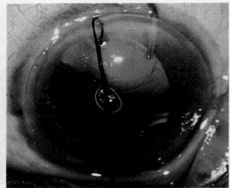

Figure 2. Deepening of the anterior chamber and pushing back hyaloid face with Healon.

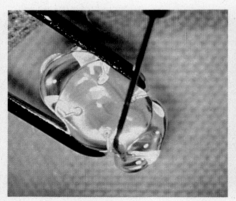

Figure 3. The coating of the intraocular lens before insertion.

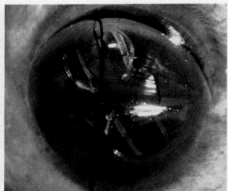

Figure 4. The engagement of the inferior pupil with the inferior loops of the lens.

86

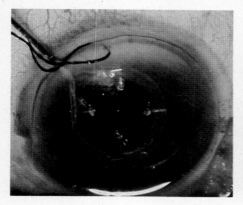

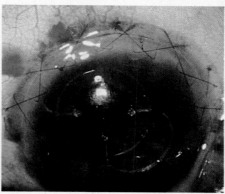

Figure 5. Superior loops engaged, some Healon now washed out of anterior chamber.

Figure 6. Wound closure using a running suture (note lustrous cornea kept moist by Healon).

must now make sure that both posterior loops are behind the iris and both anterior loops are in front. Once the lens is properly positioned, 1–2 cc of acetylcholine (Miochol) is injected into the anterior chamber. The acetylcholine will almost instantly constrict the pupil, bringing its edges around the four posts of the posterior loops and forcing the pupil to take on a square configuration. One to two cc of Carbechol (Miostat) is now instilled into the anterior chamber to maintain miosis. The presence of Healon does not slow down the effects of the miotics significantly. If any blood is trapped between lens and vitreous face, it should be gently irrigated from the eye (Figs. 1–5).

Wound Closure

The surgeon now closes the wound in his or her accustomed way. Once the wound is closed, balanced salt solution is introduced into the anterior chamber via a fine cannula. Care must be taken to keep the cannula anterior to the lens. As the saline is gently pumped into the chamber, some Healon will exit between the sutures. Not all the Healon need be replaced by physiologic saline. However, many surgeons feel that removal of some of the Healon at this time will prevent a transient, postoperative rise in intraocular pressure (Fig. 6).

Healon Related Postoperative Glaucoma

Use of Healon has been noted to produce transient postoperative rises in the intraocular pressure in some cases. On very rare occasions, pressures over 50 mm Hg have been recorded. Why does this occur?

Experiments by Berson et al. (5) in Boston have shed some light on this problem. Using enucleated human eyes perfused with Ringer's lactate solution, the facility of outflow was measured in eyes in which the anterior chamber was filled with Healon as well as in control eyes. For the first 12 hours after initiation of the experiment, the facility of outflow in the Healon-treated eyes decreased by about 50%. Irrigation of the Healon after complete chamber filling with Healon still decreased facility of outflow, but to a lesser degree. From these and other experiments, we conclude that the sodium hyaluronate sticks to the trabecular meshwork. In time, the material slowly extrudes through the pores of the meshwork. However, it leaves the eye at a slower rate than aqueous humor. Other events related to surgery—exudate and/or blood in the anterior chamber, zonular fragments digested by enzyme, release of iris pigment, tight suturing (6), limbal incisions (7)—may each impede aqueous outflow. It appears that Healon's presence in the trabecular meshwork may amplify the effects of any of the above during the first postoperative week. These effects may all be balanced by a postoperative decrease in aqueous production, and no glaucoma develops. However, transient glaucoma will ensue if the above effects combine with an early return of normal aqueous secretion.

A number of regimens have been recommended to prevent the transient glaucoma. Professor Draeger of Germany recommends use of intravenous diamox during the surgery followed by 125 mg orally t.i.d. during the immediate postoperative period. Jaffee and coworkers recommend irrigating the Healon from the anterior chamber at the end of the operation. Other surgeons feel that by avoiding tight suturing, excess Healon may leak out of the incision during the immediate postoperative period and normalize the pressure.

For more information on Healon-related elevated intraocular pressure, the reader is referred to Chapter 18.

ACKNOWLEDGMENT

The authors wish to thank the editor and publisher of the *Annals of Ophthalmology* for allowing publication of some of the material in this chapter.

REFERENCES

1. Miller, D., Stegmann, R. Use of sodium hyaluronate in human IOL implantation. *Ann. Ophthalmol.* 13:811, 1981.

2. Jaffe, N.S., Galin, M.A., Hirschman, H., Clayman, H.M. *Pseudophakos.* St. Louis, C.V. Mosby, 1978, p. 35.

3. Arzeno, G., Miller, D. Sphincter damage to pupillary stretch. (in progress)

4. Percival, S.P.B. Results after intracapsular extraction: The atonic pupil. *Ophthalmic Surg.* 8:138, 1977.

5. Berson, F.G., Epstein, D.L., Patterson, M.M. Obstruction of outflow facility by sodium hyaluronate in post-mortem enucleated eyes. ARVO Abstracts. *Invest. Ophthalmol. Vis. Sci.* 20:(March suppl.)119, 1981.

6. Campbell, D.G. The acute pressure rise following cataract extraction: Relation to complications and a new cause, sutural deformation. American Academy of Ophthalmologists Meeting, Atlanta, 1981.

7. Rothkoff, L., Biedner, B., Blumenthal, M. The effect of corneal section on early increased intraocular pressure after cataract extraction. *Am. J. Ophthalmol.* 85:337, 1978.

8. Draeger, J. Personal communication, Zurich, 1981.

7

Use of Healon in the Implantation of the Posterior Chamber Lens

Robert Stegmann

David Miller

As one reviews the history of cataract surgery, it becomes clear that the extracapsular mode of extraction has been used to break new ground on two important occasions. Jacques Daviel, a French ophthalmologist, performed the first modern type of cataract extraction in 1756 using an extracapsular technique (1). He made a large inferior limbal incision and, after a radial iridotomy and capsulotomy, spatulated the hard nucleus out of the eye "from below." No sutures were used for closure, and on the twentieth postoperative day, the patient was able to resolve fine details with a magnifying glass. A little over 200 years later, Harold Ridley, an English ophthalmologist, successfully implanted the first intraocular lens (2). Ridley employed an extracapsular technique for the cataract extraction and then inserted a biconvex plastic lens, weighing 112 mg in air, into the posterior chamber. Although the refracting power of that original lens was a bit too strong, the patient saw well with spectacles and tolerated the intraocular lens well. The posterior chamber lens has been modified and improved many times since its introduction in the autumn of 1949. The present versions of the lens weigh about $^1/_{10}$ of the original, have finely polished optics, high powers of resolution, and fit more easily into the posterior chamber. In the hands of an experienced surgeon, the posterior chamber lens may have a number of advantages over the other lens designs. Because of its position behind the iris, it produces little glare from the lens edge, allows free mobility of the pupil, has an improved cosmetic appearance, induces almost no magnification, and produces a minimum of endophthalmodonesis. In the postoperative period it seems to be associated with a low incidence of cystoid macular edema (3,4,5). Of course, posterior chamber lenses also have certain disadvantages. The lens is difficult to remove. If placed in the ciliary sulcus, it occasionally drifts inferiorly, producing monocular diplopia. The lens may also erode into the iris or ciliary body (6). Finally, a combination of the presence of the implant and an extracapsular extraction is associated with a 20–50% opacification of the posterior capsule (7,8,9).

The use of Healon can also facilitate the implantation of a posterior chamber lens. For example, Healon is helpful in protecting the corneal endothelium during implantation. Because of its viscosity, a stream of Healon directed at the edge of the pupil can give the surgeon an extra millimeter or two of pupillary dilation during the surgery. A jet of Healon can separate the leaves of the anterior capsule from the posterior allowing easier implantation within the capsule. Healon can also be used to preserve the anterior vitreous face during a posterior capsulotomy. Finally, Healon can be used to maintain the anterior chamber and keep the implant away from the endothelial surface in the event that a large window must be cut in a postoperative pupillary membrane. What follows is a step-by-step description of a posterior chamber lens implantation. Interspersed throughout the description will be headings introduced by an asterisk. These sections describe how the use of Healon improves the results of the surgery.

IMPLANTATION OF POSTERIOR CHAMBER LENS USING HEALON

Preliminary Considerations

We will assume that the surgeon has moved smoothly through the various steps of an extracapsular cataract extraction and has reached the stage at which all the nuclear and cortical material has been removed from the eye.

*Lens and Chamber Preparation

A small mound of Healon is placed on the superior conjunctiva, and the posterior chamber lens to be implanted is nestled within the mound. This mound imprisonment of the lens coats the lens and loops and will allow the surgeon to grasp the lens easily at the appropriate moment. The anterior chamber is now filled with Healon. The posterior capsule should be pushed into a mild concave configuration with a few gentle jets of Healon. If the pupil is not maximally dilated, the surgeon may enlarge the pupil 1–2 mm by directing a jet of Healon at the pupillary margin. In order to make room for the loops within the capsular bag, the cannula tip should be placed either through the iridectomy or along the pupil edge and a jet used to lift the anterior capsular leaves from the posterior capsule.

Implantation

The lens is picked up with a smooth, nontoothed forceps (such as the McPherson-Kelman forceps) by grasping the superior loop near the lens optic. The corneal lip is lifted with a fine toothed forceps by the surgeon and the implant slid into the anterior chamber, angled so as to just slip underneath the inferior iris. The lens will nestle in between anterior and posterior leaves of the capsule. Slight inferior pressure on the lens will produce mild creases in the posterior capsule, assuring proper placement. At this stage, the cornea and the superior lens loop are released. The open end of the superior loop is then grasped with the forceps. With his other hand, the surgeon introduces a 30-gauge cannula attached to the Healon syringe through a port at 3 o'clock, the lens is guided, and the loop is bent and brought into the anterior chamber until it will just slide under the superior pupillary margin and fit under the superior iris. If any difficulty is encountered, the upper iris segment may be pulled over the upper loop with a blunt iris hook, while the implant is held back with a fine repositor. Once it is posterior to the iris, the loop is released and allowed to spring back to its normal size and guided to the capsule periphery between anterior and posterior capsule. If the lens is not perfectly centered, it can be positioned by the fine cannula. Any blood captured between lens and posterior capsule should be irrigated from the eye before wound closure (Figs. 1–7).

*Posterior Capsulotomy

A hooked 30-gauge needle is now attached to the Healon syringe and brought through the iridectomy and along the posterior surface of the implant until the center of the pupil is reached. A small nick is made in the posterior capsule. A gentle jet of Healon is now injected through the small nick in order to push the vitreous face posteriorly. The nick

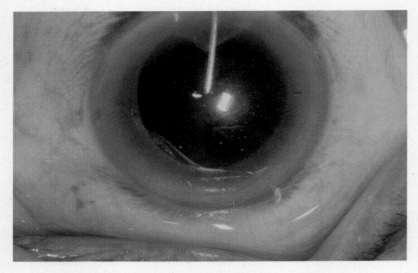

Figure 1. Deepening of anterior chamber with Healon.

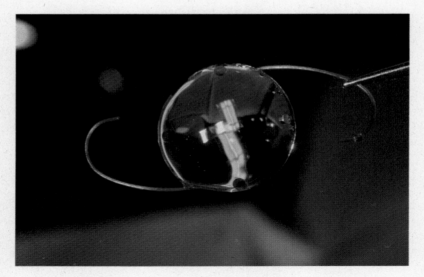

Figure 2. The coating of the intraocular lens before insertion.

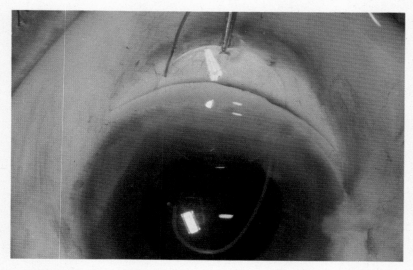

Figure 3. Direct inferior haptic towards inferior ciliary sulcus.

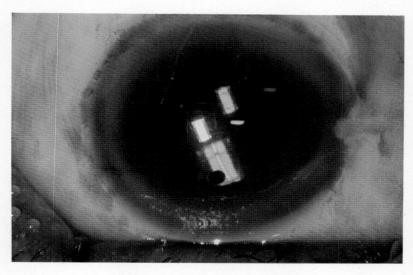

Figure 4. Inferior haptic in place.

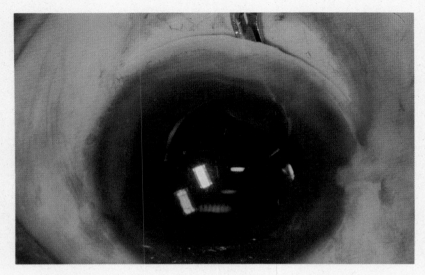

Figure 5. Positioning superior haptic in superior sulcus.

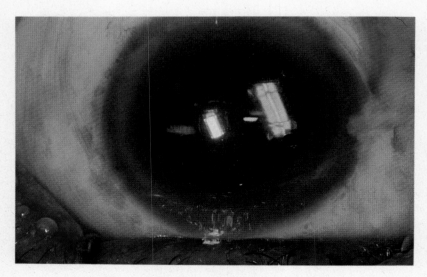

Figure 6. Posterior chamber lens in place.

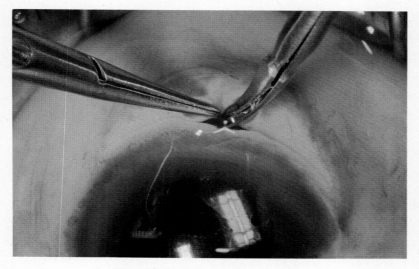

Figure 7. Peripheral iridectomy.

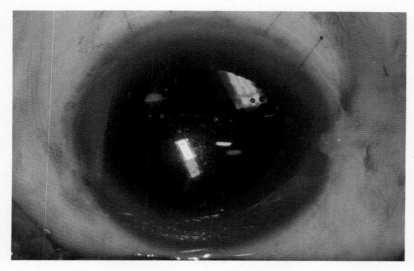

Figure 8. Sutures in place.

can now be safely enlarged to a few millimeters without rupturing the vitreous face.

Wound Closure

The wound is now closed with a series of interrupted 9-0 or 10-0 nylon sutures. The free ends are cut with a razor blade on the knot and the sutures pulled beneath the surface of the wound (Fig. 8).

Additional Measures

At this time, subconjunctival corticosteroids and antibiotics may be injected if desired by the surgeon. A monocular dressing is then taped in place protected by a plastic or metal shield.

REFERENCES

1. Duke Elder, S. *System of Ophthalmology*. St. Louis, C.V. Mosby, 1969, vol. 11, p. 248.
2. Perritt, R.A. Intraocular lens implantation from Ridley to the present: My 25 years experience. *Int. Ophthalmol. Clin.* 19:11, 1979.
3. Binkhorst, C.D., Kats, A., Tjan, T.T. et al. Intracapsular vs. extracapsular surgery. *Trans. Am. Acad. Ophthalmol. and Otolaryngol.* 83:120, 1976.
4. Jaffe, N.S. Results of intracapsular implant surgery, in *Symposium on Cataracts, Trans. New Orleans Acad. Ophth.* St. Louis, C.V. Mosby, 1979, p. 310.
5. Kratz, R.P., Mazzocco, T.R., Davidson, B., Colvard, D.M. The Shearing intraocular lens: A report of 1000 cases. *Am. Intraocular Implant Soc. J.* 7:55, 1981.
6. Olson, R.J., Morgan, K.S., Kolodner, H. The Shearing intraocular lens: Where does it go and what does it do in the eye? *Ophthalmology* 87:668, 1980.
7. Emery, J.H. Opacified posterior capsule/retro-implant membranes, in Emery, J.H. (ed): *Current Concepts in Cataract Surgery*. St. Louis, C.V. Mosby, 1978, pp. 433–437.
8. Sinskey, R.M., Cain, W. The posterior capsule and phacoemulsification. *Am. Intraocular Implant Soc. J.* 4:206, 1978.
9. Worst, J.G.F. Extracapsular surgery and lens implantation. *Ophthalmic Surgery* 8:33, 1977.

8

Secondary Intraocular Lens Implantation Using Healon

Robert Stegmann

David Miller

Introduction

A number of years ago, the term *20/20 cripple* (1) was coined for the spectacle-corrected aphake who saw the eye chart clearly in the doctor's office, but had difficulty functioning in a real world distorted by aphakic spectacles. Contact lenses helped change that for many aphakes. However, there are still many who cannot master the insertion and removal aspects because of arthritis, tremors, or the anxiety associated with placing a device in one's eye. Continuous wear contact lenses may help many of these patients. However, there is about a 15% failure rate associated with these lenses (2,3). Is it reasonable to consider secondary intraocular lens (IOL) implantation in these cases? Certainly the optical advantages are obvious, and very little maintenance is involved. But, what of the risks? The more remote complications would include endophthalmitis, expulsive hemorrhage, epithelialization of the anterior chamber, and death related to anesthesia (4). Common complications include about a 20% vitreous loss (5), a 5–20% incidence of cystoid macular edema (5,6,7,8), and further endothelial cell loss.

The use of the viscoelastic sodium-hyaluronate (9,10) (Healon®, Pharmacia Labs, NJ) should give the ophthalmologist a safe way of protecting the corneal endothelium, maintaining a deep anterior chamber during instrument manipulation and pushing the vitreous face behind the iris, and, thus, performing secondary implantation in a safer manner.

Table 1. Intraocular Pressure
Associated With Secondary Implantation

Number	Average IOP ± S.D.
Preoperative	
20	14.3 mm Hg ± 3.6
Postoperative	
20	10.4 mm Hg ± 3.3

In order to evaluate this hypothesis, we studied 20 patients who received a secondary implant using Healon at surgery.

All 20 patients were unilateral aphakes. In every case, a combination of the patients' need for binocular vision and their inability to succeed with contact lenses motivated them to request the implantation. The patients ranged from 35 to 55 years of age. The initial cataract extraction had been performed from six months to four years prior to secondary implantation. Seventeen were intracapsular and three were extracapsular extractions. Twenty-four hours before surgery, the following tests were performed on the eye to be operated on: best spectacle corrected visual acuity, intraocular pressure, corneal thickness measurements, and endothelial cell counts. On the first postoperative day, intraocular pressure measurements and corneal thickness measurements were obtained. At the end of the fourth postoperative week, best corrected visual acuity was recorded and central corneal endothelial cell counts remeasured.

The Binkhorst 4-loop pupillary plane lens was used in 15 cases, the Binkhorst 2-loop iridocapsular lens in two cases, and the Shearing posterior chamber lens in three cases.

Table 1 compares the average preoperative and first day postoperative intraocular pressure. Note that there is no significant postoperative rise in pressure.

Table 2. Corneal Thickness Associated with
Secondary Implantation

Number	Average Thickness (mm) ± S.D.
Preoperative	
20	0.51 mm ± .012
Postoperative	
20	0.53 mm ± .014

Table 3. Corneal Endothelial Cell Counts Associated with Secondary Implantation

Number	Average Cell Count ± S.D.	Average Cell Loss	Percent Cell Loss
Preoperative 20	2046 cells/mm² ± 579		
		159	7.1%
Postoperative 20	1887 cells/mm² ± 535		

Table 2 compares the average preoperative and first day postoperative corneal thickness. There is no significant postoperative increase in corneal thickness.

Table 3 compares the average preoperative and four week postoperative endothelial cell count. An average of a 7.1% decrease in endothelial cells had occurred as the result of surgery.

Table 4 compares the best corrected visual acuity preoperatively and at one month after surgery. The $1/2$ line loss after surgery may be related to the decrease of magnification introduced when the intraocular lens replaced the spectacle.

No vitreous loss was noted in any case.

No evidence of cystoid macular edema was noted one month after surgery. However, this latter observation must be evaluated with the understanding that this patient population rarely develops cystoid macular disease.

Follow-up on these patients has been between six and 24 months.

The postoperative courses of the patients in the study have been uniformly smooth, and, in a few cases where iris fluorescein angiography was performed on the third postoperative day, the amount of leakage was considerably less than the average leakage in a primary implantation.

Table 4. Best Corrected Visual Acuity Associated with Secondary Implantation

Number	Visual Acuity (Average)
Preoperative 20	20/25
Postoperative 20	20/30 − 3

What follows is a step-by-step description of a secondary implantation. Interspersed throughout the description will be headings introduced by an asterisk. These sections describe how Healon improves the results of the surgery.

SECONDARY IOL IMPLANTATIONS

Preliminary Considerations

After an intracapsular cataract extraction, an anterior chamber lens or a pupillary plane lens is generally used for a secondary implantation. Although, the study reported the results with pupillary plane lenses, we have come to learn that use of anterior chamber lenses have a higher success rate. Therefore we will describe the procedure using the anterior chamber lens. The surgeon may use his or her usual prepping and draping techniques, mode of anesthesia, and method of ocular massage. A favored lid speculum is then placed in the eye. A muscle hook may be used to sweep the fornices in order to see that there are no pressure contacts between globe and speculum. A superior rectus stay suture is then inserted for globe immobilization.

Incision

Although a standard limbal incision under a flap can be used for secondary lens implantation, the authors used a corneal incision in this series. Therefore, the technique using a corneal section will be described.

A 2–3 mm section, 1 mm corneal to the limbus, is made with a sharp blade at 12 o'clock. A puff of aqueous announces entrance into the anterior chamber.

*Chamber Filling

The Healon syringe is armed with a 30-gauge cannula. The cannula tip is inserted into the incision. At the time Healon is introduced into the chamber, the aqueous simultaneously leaves through the edge of the incision. Enough viscoelastic Healon is introduced to push the vitreous face and iris into a flat configuration. The filling of the chamber should be gradual with the cannula slowly advancing toward the inferior limbus, almost pushing the vitreous back in units.

*Lens Implantation

The incision is enlarged to 6 mm to allow entry of the anterior chamber lens. The superior loop is grasped with a toothless forceps and the front surface of the lens coated with Healon. The inferior loop is then slipped into the incision and the lens slid over the surface of the iris until the inferior loop engages the inferior angle. The lens is gently rocked to free it from any possible iris tuck. The superior loop is now placed under the lip of the wound (Figs. 1–6).

Wound Closure

The corneal incision is then closed with three or four interrupted 10-0 nylon sutures. Subconjunctival steriods and antibiotics are then given.

*Final Precautions

Since some patients demonstrate a transient postoperative rise in intra-ocular pressure after Healon usage, the following is recommended to prevent such a complication. After the wound is tightly closed, a 30-

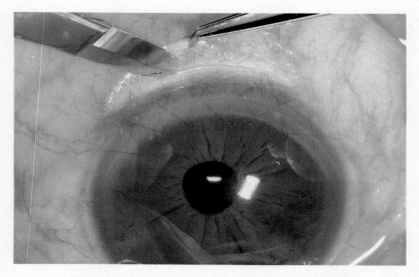

Figure 1. Mobilizing limbal based conjunctival flap.

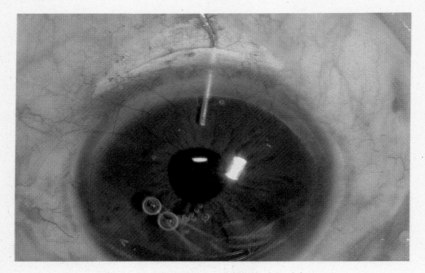

Figure 2. Appearance of limbal incision.

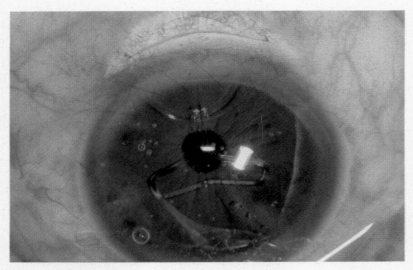

Figure 3. Deepening the anterior chamber with Healon after small entry puncture.

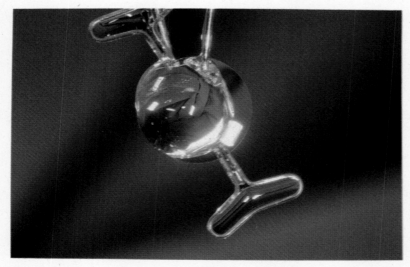

Figure 4. The coating of the intraocular lens with Healon before insertion.

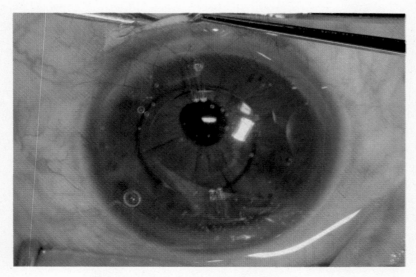

Figure 5. Implantation of anterior chamber lens.

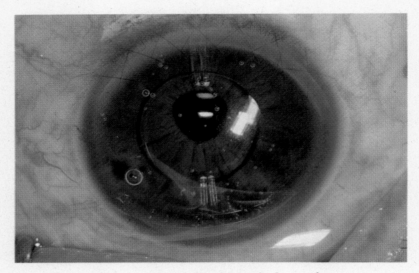

Figure 6. Wound closed at end of procedure.

gauge cannula, attached to a bottle or syringe of physiologic saline, is introduced into the anterior chamber at the edge of the wound. Some saline is advanced into the chamber. This maneuver should drive out most of the Healon present in the chamber and should prevent any significant transient rise in intraocular pressure. If a pressure elevation is encountered postoperatively, local timolol drops or systemic acetazolamide given for a few days will bring the pressure under control.

ACKNOWLEDGMENT

The authors wish to thank the publisher and editor of the *Journal of Ocular Therapeutics and Surgery* for allowing the publication of some of the material in this chapter.

REFERENCES

1. Sloane, A. Visual acuity is not a number. *Arch. Ophthalmol.* 68:440, 1962.
2. Slatt, B., Stein, H.A. Complications of prolonged wear hydrogel lenses. *Contact and Intraocular Lens Med. J.* 5:82, 1979.

3. Freeman, M.I., Chandler, J.W. Extended wear of aphakic contact lenses. *Contact and Intraocular Lens Med. J.* 5:76, 1979.

4. Burde, A.M. Complications in intraocular lens implantation, in Waltman, S.R., Krupin, T. (eds): *Complications in Ophthalmic Surgery.* Philadelphia, J.B. Lippincott, 1980, p. 94.

5. Azar, R.F. Secondary implantation of intraocular lenses. *Ann. Ophthalmol.* 10:658, 1978.

6. Choyce, D.P. The Choyce Mark VIII anterior chamber implant: Primary and secondary implantation compared. *Ophthalmic. Surg.* 8:49, 1977.

7. Shammas, H.J.F., Milkie, C.F. Primary vs. secondary insertion of anterior chamber lenses. *Am. Intraocular Implant Soc. J.* 5:141, 1979.

8. Hardenburgh, F.E. Secondary intraocular lens implantation. *Ophthalmic Surg.* 8:70, 1977.

9. Miller D., Stegmann, R. Use of Na-hyaluronate in anterior segment eye surgery. *Am. Intraocular Implant Soc. J.* 6:13, 1980.

10. Miller, D., Stegmann, R. Secondary intraocular lens implantation using Na-hyaluronate. *J. Ocular Ther. and Surg.* (In press.)

9
Intraocular Lens Removal Using Healon

Robert Stegmann

David Miller

Introduction

Bioprostheses are, unfortunately, not always accepted by the body, and, on occasion, may have to be removed. It also follows that the inventor or developer of the bioprosthesis is usually the first to see the occasion of an incompatibility between the prostheses and the body, and the first to surgically remove the device. For example, the pioneering orthopedic surgeons who initially replaced frozen arthritic hip joints with artificial ones were forced to remove every one of them after they became loose (1). In the field of intraocular lens, the pioneering developer must have been witness to some serious incompatibilities, for he reported removing 15% of those he implanted (2). Of course, the lenses of today are more carefully made, and the incidence of lens removal has dropped to about 1.5% (3). Today's lenses are lighter, smoother, more precisely polished, and more apt to be free of contaminants and foreign material. However, there still are instances when the implant should be removed. There seem to be three general categories where the need for lens removal will occur. The first category contains cases in which the lens is rubbing, irritating, or on the verge of rubbing or irritating one of the delicate structures of the eye. This category would include impending or real corneal touch, chronic uveitis, the development of rubeosis irides after implantation, events causing chronic and severe cystoid macular edema, chronic glaucoma, and iris erosion. A subgroup of patients would include those in which the postoperative inflammation has produced adhesions to the lens and the lens has become grossly decentered. The second category is the presence of endophthalmitis. Such cases are often due to the implantation of a contaminated lens. The third and last category includes those cases with a history of repeated dislocations of the lens. After a number of trying and anxiety evoking repositions of the lens, either doctor or patient may suggest that the lens should come out.

Once a decision to remove a lens is made, the question of lens exchange must be addressed. If the reason for the incompatibility between the lens and the eye can be identified, that is, lens incorrectly positioned and rubbing against corneal endothelium, then a second question must be raised. Is there available a new lens, perhaps of a different design, that will avoid the original problem? If the answer is a theoretical yes, then a third and somewhat embarrassing question must be asked. Does the surgeon have the ability and experience to place the new lens correctly? If the answers to all three questions are strongly affirmative, then lens exchange after lens removal is the proper course. When facing such a difficult series of questions, the venerable observation, "No man is an island unto himself," should be considered. If the solution is not totally obvious, outside consultation should be sought.

The technique of lens removal centers on a basic theme: The implant must not damage the corneal endothelium as it is being removed. Before the advent of Healon viscosurgery, this usually meant that the lens had to be mobilized, that is, suture or fixation clip opened or synechiae lysed in a closed eye in which an air bubble held the lens away from the endothelium. Such an approach involved the clever use of fine hooks and spatulas, which had to be inserted into the eye through small incisions without disturbing the air bubble. With Healon, the closed eye approach can be abandoned because Healon will keep the implant from the corneal endothelium in the face of a large incision, as well as keep the structures of the anterior chamber in the proper anatomic relationship.

In the description to follow, the steps in which Healon is used will be introduced by an asterisk.

REMOVAL OF AN IOL

Preliminary Considerations

The surgeon may use his or her usual method of preparation and draping of the patient as well as the accustomed mode of anesthesia, along with the usual lid speculum placement and superior rectus stay suture insertion. In the removal of pupillary plane and posterior chamber lenses, preoperative maximal pupillary dilation using six applications of 10% phenylephrine and 1% Mydriacyl or 1% cyclopentolate should be given.

*Incision

Aside from an eye with a chronically dislocated lens, an eye in which an implant necessitates removal is an irritated and markedly inflamed eye. Thus, increased bleeding during the surgery is to be expected. Therefore, it has been recommended that, whenever possible, a clear corneal incision be made to minimize bleeding (3) and to keep the events taking place within the eye highly visible. A groove should be made just corneal to the limbal vessels with a rounded knife for about 3–4 hours of the clock. The groove and incision should be centered over an area of intact iris. In most cases, this will be at the 12 o'clock position. The groove is then punctured with a razor blade knife. After a puff of aqueous is seen at the puncture site, Healon is introduced into the anterior chamber through a fine cannula. The chamber should be completely filled so that there is a thick blanket of Healon between the lens and the cornea. The incision is then enlarged with corneal scissors to about 8 mm.

Implant Mobilization

If a suture is holding the lens to the iris, it should be cut with fine scissors and removed from the eye. If a stave has engaged the lens, the lens must be stabilized with a spatula or forceps and the stave opened with a toothless forceps. Now a careful inspection must be made in order to see if adhesions are present between lens and iris, lens and vitreous, or lens and incision site. Any adhesion found must be gently lysed with a fine cyclodialysis spatula. The lens is now grasped with a smooth forceps (e.g., Kelman forceps) and slid out of the wound. Normally the posterior lip of the sclera will have to be depressed with a spatula or forceps. The exiting lens should be irrigated with a stream of physiologic saline to help differentiate adherent vitreous from adherent Healon. A string of Healon will quickly dissolve under the barrage of the jet, whereas vitreous will remain adherent and stringy. If vitreous adhesions are present, they must be cut. Free vitreous in the anterior chamber should be removed using a vitrectomy technique so that no vitreous is present to adhere to the wound edges. Anterior chamber lenses are easiest to remove because of their uniplanar structure and their position in the anterior chamber. An easy method of removing these anterior chamber lenses is to grasp the posterior corneal lip with a forceps and pull toward the surgeon while placing a spatula under one of the superior feet and gently tip it upward. The lens will often simply slide out of the incision. Occasionally, a smooth forceps will be needed to grasp a foot close to the wound and gently rotate the lens out of the wound.

For removal of a posterior chamber lens that has become adherent to the capsule or the ciliary sulcus, a more conservative tact is in order. The objective is to remove the lens but let part of the loop remain. Lysis of adhesions between lens and iris and lens and capsule may be attempted with jets of Healon. If such jets fail to break the adhesions, then a spatula or fine scissors should be tried. Once the lens is free, the superior pupil is retracted as far as possible and the loop cut close to the pupillary margin. The superior lens is then grasped with a smooth forceps and gently maneuvered into the anterior chamber. If resistance from adhesions to the inferior loop are felt or seen, a small but sturdy blunt-tipped scissors is run along the loop until the scissor tips are just in view, and this loop is cut. The lens, under a blanket of Healon, is now slid out of the incision. If a dense pupillary membrane is present after lens removal, Healon will be of great help in dissecting out a window in the membrane. A small nick is first made in the membrane. Healon is then injected through the membrane in order to push back the vitreous face. A square window is now cut in the pupillary portion of the membrane using very fine scissors or an automated membrane cutter. See Figures 1–11 for

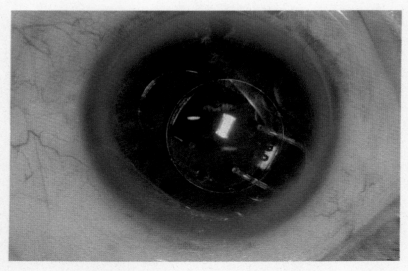

Figure 1. Chronically dislocated pupillary plane lens in anterior chamber.

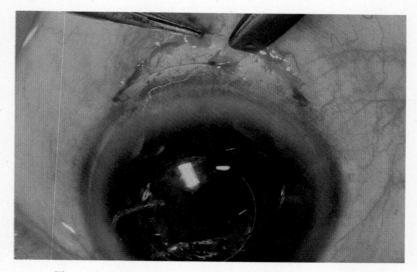

Figure 2. Corneal-scleral incision with fornix-based flap.

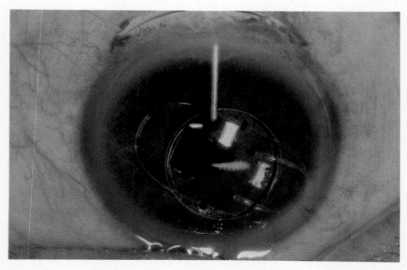

Figure 3. Deepening anterior chamber with Healon (to protect endothelium).

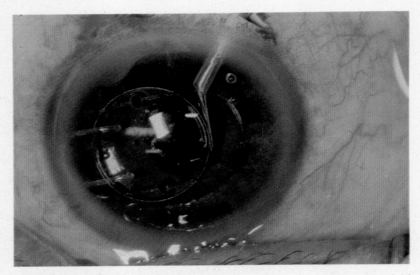

Figure 4. Cutting of offending synnechiae (with maintenance of hyaloid face).

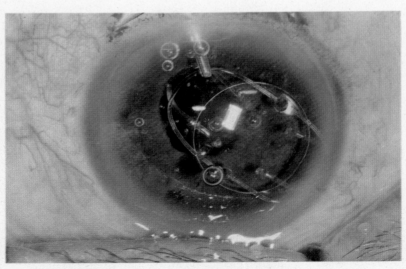

Figure 5. Grasp superior haptic with fine forceps.

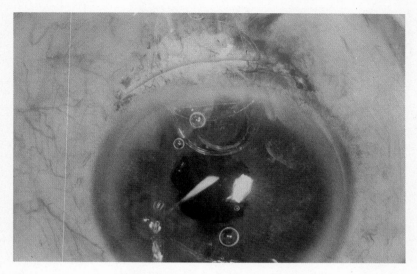

Figure 6. Sliding implant out of incision.

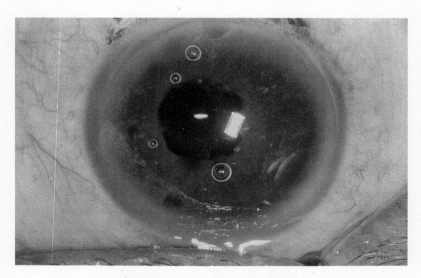

Figure 7. Chamber reformed with Healon.

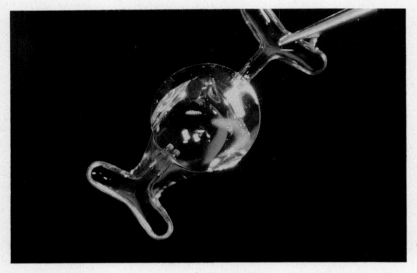

Figure 8. Healon-coated anterior chamber lens to be used as secondary implant.

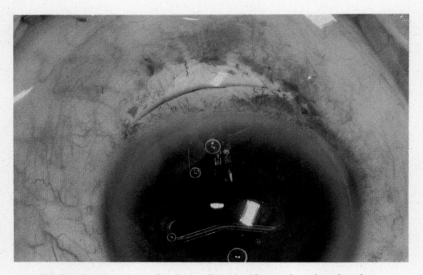

Figure 9. Insertion of inferior haptic of anterior chamber lens.

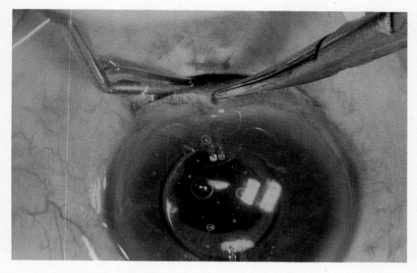

Figure 10. Positioning of superior haptic under scleral shelf.

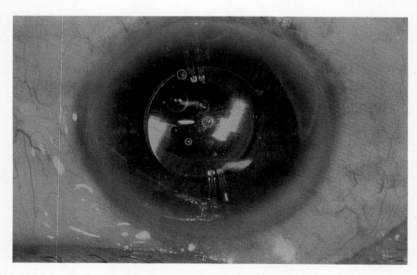

Figure 11. Sutures in place.

technique of removing chronically dislocated lenses and implanting secondary anterior chamber lens.

Wound Closure

Closure can be accomplished with interrupted 9-0 or 10-0 nylon sutures. Care should be taken to deepen the chamber after closure with air or saline.

Postoperative Medication

Because these eyes, in general, have been chronically irritated eyes, one can anticipate that the postoperative course will be stormy. Therefore, we recommend the use of subconjunctival corticosteroids at the close of surgery. During the postoperative period, treatment should include the use of corticosteroids and mydriatic drops.

REFERENCES

1. Judet, J., Judet, R. The use of an artificial femoral head for arthroplasty of the hip joint. *J. Bone Joint Surg.* 323:166, 1950.
2. Jaffe, N.S., Galin, M.A., Hirschman, H., Clayman, H.M. *Pseudophakos.* St. Louis, C.V. Mosby, 1978, p. 37.
3. Sheppard, D.D. Indications for intraocular lens removal. *Ophthalmic Surg.* 8:144, 1977.

10

Corneal Transplantation Using Healon

Robert Stegmann

David Miller

Introduction

It seems amazing that long before the introduction of the slit lamp and operating microscope, Leber (1,2) knew of the presence of the single, transparent layer of cells that line the back of the cornea. In 1873, he showed that if he rubbed the back of a bovine cornea, it became water-logged much sooner than a control cornea. Nevertheless, work on the role of the endothelium in corneal transplantation moved slowly until after World War II. In the early 1950s, Stocker (3) and Leigh (4) elegantly showed the importance of handling the donor endothelium delicately if a clear graft was to be achieved. As the eminence of endothelial integrity in corneal transplantation rose, improved storage techniques (5) were developed. The 1950s and the 1960s were also times in which finer needles and forceps (6) and finally microscopic control (7) were introduced. By the 1970s, many surgeons intuitively sensed the importance of not allowing the endothelium to touch any surface, including the iris and lens of the recipient. Therefore, such techniques as air bubble introduction into the chamber (8), soft contact lenses draped over the wound edge during suturing (9), and use of oversized donor buttons (10) were developed. However, actual proof of the preservation of corneal endothelial cells, using these techniques, had to await the development of the endothelial camera (11,12). Then, for the first time, cell loss following successful keratoplasty was measured (11). Studies at that time also showed increased endothelial loss if the donor button touched recipient lens and iris (13). In 1977, a study was published that showed

119

that sodium hyaluronate protected the endothelium against the destructive touch of intraocular lenses during implantation into rabbit eyes (14). A second study soon followed that demonstrated that sodium hyaluronate (Healon) also preserved corneal integrity better than standard techniques in animal corneal transplantation (15). The study to be described then investigated the role of Healon in human corneal transplantation (16).

The study involved 48 patients who received corneal transplants for a spectrum of corneal disease ranging from traumatic scars through postinfection scars to degenerations. The age of the patients varied from 12 to 73 years. Forty of the patients had their corneal transplantation performed with Healon. These operations were performed between 1978 and 1980. The other eight patients, who served as controls, had their surgery performed just before the introduction of Healon.

The same experienced surgeon was involved in all 48 operations. In the Healon group, six eyes were aphakic and 34 eyes were phakic. In the control group, all eight eyes were phakic.

The age of the donor tissue ranged from 1 to 17 years and all donor tissue was used within 18 hours after the death of the donor.

The patients serving as controls, that is, those receiving surgery performed without Healon, were recalled for endothelial photography two to three years after their surgery. Endothelial counts were performed in a similar way.

Although not documented by quantitative scientific instruments, the psychological stress placed on the surgeon is significantly reduced with the knowledge that the endothelium is protected by the viscous Healon throughout the operation. Uniform suturing is also easier with the donor button held in a domelike configuration by the Healon.

As noted in Table 1, the average postoperative endothelial cell count in the 40 patients comprising the Healon group was 2738 cells/mm^2. The average endothelial cell count in the control series was 1580 cells/mm^2. Note that these are central corneal endothelial counts. These counts may not reflect the events taking place in the corneal periphery. Using

Table 1. Endothelial Cell Counts After Corneal Transplantation

	Healon Group		Control Group
No. cases	40		8
Mean	2745		1580
Standard deviation	580		727
Differences of mean		1165 cells/mm^2	
Significance of differences		0.01 level	

Student's *t* test, the difference is statistically significant at the 0.01 level.

There was no significant elevation of intraocular pressure in any of the patients in the Healon experimental group or the control group during the postoperative period.

The unsophisticated observer at surgery has no trouble appreciating how the clear viscous Healon immerses the corneal endothelium and seems to protectively cushion these cells from contact with both donor and recipient tissue. The surprising clarity of the Healon-treated cornea on the first postoperative day compared to the control eyes further attests to the usefulness of Healon.

What follows is a step-by-step description of the technique of corneal transplantation. The headings preceded by an asterisk describe the way that Healon can be used to improve the results of the operation.

CORNEAL TRANSPLANTATION USING HEALON

Preliminary Considerations

The surgeon is free to use his or her usual method of preparing and draping the patient, mode of anesthesia, and method of ocular massage. A moist gauze pad is placed over the patient's closed eye until the donor button has been prepared.

*Preparation of the Donor Cornea

The donor eye is removed from the storage bottle in the operating room. The donor eye is wrapped in sterile gauze and set on the flat surface of a sterilely draped table. An 8-mm trephine is placed over the corneal center. Trephination is continued until the anterior chamber is entered in a small area. Healon is introduced into the eye until the anterior chamber is completely filled. This will protect the donor endothelium during the removal of the button. Once the chamber is entered, the free edge of the potential donor button is grasped with fine toothed forceps, and the button removal is completed with corneal scissors. A mound of Healon is then placed in a small flat sterile dish or container and the donor button is immersed in the mound, endothelial side facing up (Figs. 1, 2, and 3).

*Trephination of Patient's Cornea

Attention is now directed to the patient's eye. The moist gauze pad is removed and a lid speculum is placed in the eye. A muscle hook is run

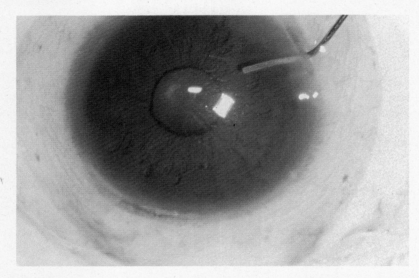

Figure 1. Inject Healon into stab incision in order to fill the anterior chamber in donor eye.

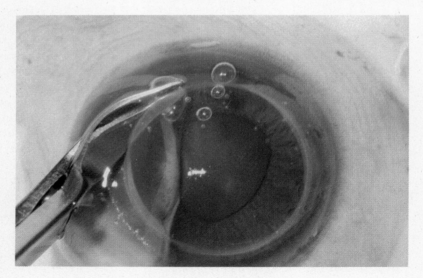

Figure 2. Cutting out donor button.

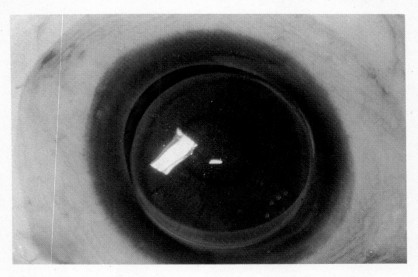

Figure 3. Donor button lying on mound of Healon in donor eye.

along the upper and lower fornices to make sure that no pressure is exerted from the speculum to the globe. An 8-mm trephine is adjusted onto the corneal center and rotated so as to just enter the anterior chamber in one small location. Healon is then injected through a cannula to fill the chamber and push the iris-lens diaphragm back. Fixation of the globe during trephination is accomplished using a tissue fixation forceps applied just off the limbus. Once the chamber is entered, excision of the pathologic corneal button is done with a fine corneal scissors, held perpendicular to the corneal surface. Any residual shelf or strands of cornea should be dissected from the sides of the opening so that the walls are relatively straight and ready to appose the sides of the donor button (Figs. 4, 5, 6, and 7)

*Further Preparation of the Patient's Eye

In cases where a cataract was present, the lens is extracted through the trephinated opening using a cryoextractor unit. If vitreous should fill the anterior chamber, an anterior vitrectomy must be performed to clear the chamber. It is also adviseable to perform a peripheral iridectomy at this point in the operation.

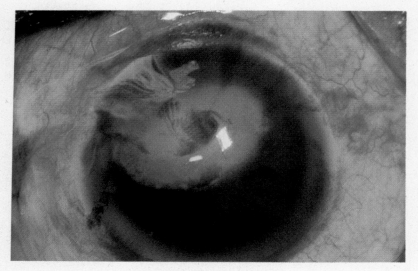

Figure 4. Diseased cornea.

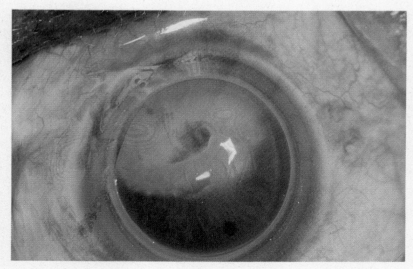

Figure 5. Trephine groove in recipient's cornea.

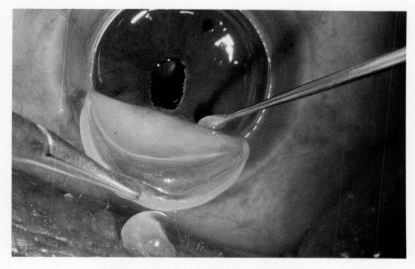

Figure 6. Cutting iridocorneal adhesion.

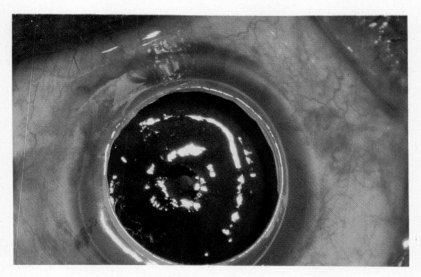

Figure 7. Removing opaque cornea.

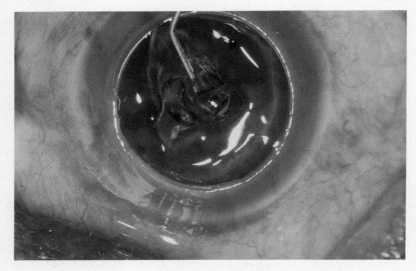

Figure 8. Placement of Healon into recipient anterior chamber.

Once the eye is ready for the donor button, the anterior chamber is filled with Healon. About 0.5 cc is used for this purpose (Fig. 8).

*Placement and Fixation of Donor Button

The donor button covered with Healon is gently grasped with fine toothed forceps, avoiding endothelial touch, fitted into the trephined opening, and allowed to settle onto the bed of Healon. Using 10-0 monofilament nylon, four fixation sutures (cardinal sutures) are placed in an interrupted fashion in the four corneal quadrants. In the case of the aphakic eye with a bulging vitreous face, once the four cardinal sutures are tightly tied, more Healon is gently introduced into the anterior chamber. This maneuver tends to push the vitreous face back. A running suture averaging six bites per quadrant and of $^1/_2$ to $^3/_4$ corneal thickness is then completed. Each bit should be taken at least 2 mm on either side of the incision. The tension of the suture is then adjusted so that wound apposition is as uniform as possible for 360°. A triple throw knot then unites the two loose ends of the running suture. Two single throws make the knot permanent. If some Healon has been squeezed out of the anterior chamber during suturing, more Healon is introduced so as to always maintain a domed configuration of the new cornea (Figs. 9, 10, and 11).

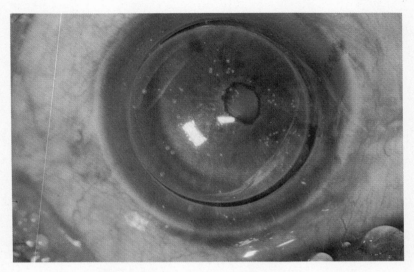

Figure 9. Transfer donor button onto recipient eye.

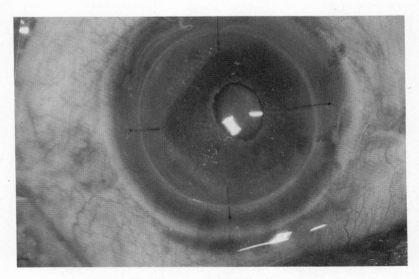

Figure 10. Placement of cardinal sutures.

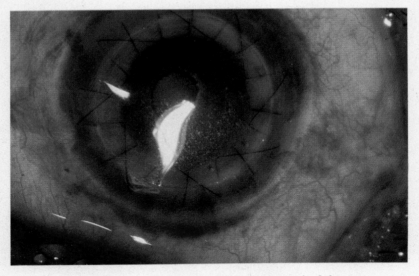

Figure 11. Running sutures in place at the end of the case.

Final Precautions

At this point, a fine cannula attached to a syringe filled with balanced salt solution is introduced into the anterior chamber, and some Healon is forced out of the wound. This maneuver is designed to avoid a transient elevation in intraocular pressure after the surgery.

Final Medication

At the close of the procedure, 0.1–0.5 cc of corticosteroid and 0.1 cc of antibiotic are injected into the subconjunctival space. A double eye pad and protective shield are then taped over the patient's eye.

ACKNOWLEDGMENT

The authors wish to thank the publisher and editor of the *Journal of Ocular Therapeutics and Surgery* for allowing the publication of some of the material in this chapter.

REFERENCES

1. Leber, T. Studien ueber den Fluessigkeitswechel im Auge. *Graefes Arch. Ophth.* 19, Abt. 2:87, 1873.

2. Wagenmann, A. Experimentelle Untersuchungen zur Frage der Keratoplastik. *Graefes Arch. Ophth.* Abt. 1:211, 1888.

3. Stocker, F.W. *The Endothelium of the Cornea and Its Clinical Implications* Springfield, Il. Charles C. Thomas, 1971, p. 156.

4. Leigh, A.G. *Corneal Transplantation.* Oxford, Blackwell Scientific Publications, 1966, p. 50.

5. Stocker, F.W. *The Endothelium of the Cornea and Its Clinical Implications.* Springfield, Il., Charles C. Thomas, 1971, p. 156.

6. Rycroft, P.V. (ed). *Microsurgery and Keratoplasty in Cornea Plastic Surgery.* Oxford, Pergamon Press, 1969, p. 341.

7. Troutman, R.C. Microsurgery for keratoplasty. *Int. Ophthalmol. Clin.* 10:297, 1970.

8. Jones, B.R., Rice, N.S.C. The avoidance of damage to the corneal endothelium in penetrating keratoplasty, in Rycroft, P.V. (ed): *Corneo-Plastic Surgery.* Oxford, Pergamon Press, 1969, p. 307.

9. Kramer, S.G., Stewart, H.L. Maintenance of the anterior chamber during penetrating keratoplasty. *Trans. Am. Acad. Ophthalmol. and Otolaryngol.* 81:794, 1976.

10. Bourne, W.M. Reduction of endothelial cell loss during phakic penetrating keratoplasty. *Am. J. Ophthalmol.* 89:787, 1980.

11. Bourne, W.M., Kaufman, H.E. The endothelium of clear corneal transplant. *Arch. Ophthalmol.* 94:1730, 1976.

12. Laing, R.A., Sandstrom, M.M., Leibowitz, H.M. In vivo photomicrography of the corneal endothelium. *Arch. Ophthalmol.* 93:143, 1975.

13. Bourne, W.M., O'Fallon, W.M. Endothelial cell loss during penetrating keratoplasty. *Am. J. Ophthalmol.* 85:760, 1978.

14. Miller, D., O'Connor, P., Williams, J. Use of Na-hyaluronate during intraocular lens implantation in rabbits. *Ophthalmic Surg.* 8:58, 1977.

15. Miller, D., Stegmann, R. Use of Na-hyaluronate in autocorneal transplantation in rabbits. *Ophthalmic Surg.* 11:19, 1980.

16. Miller, D., Stegmann, R. Use of Na-hyaluronate in corneal transplantation. *J. Ocular Ther. and Surg.* 1:28, 1981.

11

The Triple Procedure: Penetrating Keratoplasty, Cataract Extraction, and IOL Implantation Using Healon

Robert Stegmann

David Miller

Introduction

Present-day management of a patient with severe corneal disease combined with significant cataract almost epitomizes the change that has taken place in the philosophy of ophthalmic surgery. Until recently, the conservative theories of eye surgery—do the least amount of surgery at any one sitting; or the more time spent manipulating the tissues of the eye, the greater the chances for a disaster on the table—were the predominant schools of thought. Such philosophies were appropriate when our instruments of repair, the sutures and needles, were large and would themselves disrupt tissue, and we depended upon loupe magnification. Our surgical approach started to change with the introduction of microsurgical technique. The use of anti-inflammatory agents also freed us from Nature's overexuberant response to ocular trauma and has allowed us to individually titrate the healing response. Armed with the above methods, a bold challenge to the conservative school took place in the late 1960s when Katzin (1) reported a 70% success rate with simultaneous keratoplasty and cataract extraction. His work was con-

131

firmed by both Casey (2) and Kaufman (3), and the field moved closer to total surgical, visual rehabilitation. By the 1970s the implantation of an intraocular lens was combined with simultaneous keratoplasty and cataract extraction. Were we pushing our luck? Were these pioneers overstepping the bounds of reasonable management? Not at all. These pioneers reported success rates with the triple procedure that were comparable to penetrating keratoplasty alone (4–8).

One must also appreciate the social milieu in which all this was taking place. Just as all segments of our society were demanding to be heard politically, so, too, patients were demanding a higher quality of life from the doctor. Coronary bypass surgery to free them from angina, cosmetic surgery to allow patients to look as young as they felt, and joint prostheses to allow frozen joints to move were examples of medicine's response to society's new demands. Along with improving the patient's quality of life was the request to return the patient to life's mainstream as soon as possible. These two pressures clearly influenced our approach to visual rehabilitation.

It was fitting that Healon viscosurgery should also be introduced in the 1970s. All workers in the field agree that the watchword for a successful triple procedure is endothelial protection, and Healon certainly guarantees such protection. As opposed to air bubbles that may unexpectedly escape from the chamber, the viscous Healon predictably holds the tissues of the anterior segment in proper position while the surgeon deliberately goes about the business of accurate repair. However, the triple procedure is not without problems.

Because the patient's cornea may be irregular and the ultimate curvature of the transplanted cornea unpredictable, the determination of the proper power for the implant is imprecise. Our only guide is the advice of Lee and Dohlman (5), that the arbitrary use of a 19D pupillary plane lens gave satisfactory results in most cases. It might be best also to tell the patient that if the transplant develops an irregular or high astigmatism, that he or she may have to wear a contact lens or spectacles.

Is there a specific type of IOL that should be used in the triple procedure? Everyone seems to agree that rigid anterior chamber lenses cannot be fitted easily into the trephinated opening. Most studies to date report satisfactory results with the pupillary plane lens. However, Lindstrom (et al.) (9) report equally good results using an extracapsular cataract extraction and posterior chamber lens. This latter approach has the advantage of a lower incidence of vitreous loss and cystoid macular edema. These investigators also feel that the posterior capsule can be cleaned more completely through a trephine opening than through a typical cataract limbal incision, and indeed their series reports not one instance of posterior capsule opacification requiring further surgery. Thus, all but rigid anterior chamber lenses may be used in the triple procedure.

What follows is a step-by-step description of the triple procedure. The headings proceeded by an asterisk describe the way that Healon can be used to improve the results of the operation.

THE TRIPLE PROCEDURE

Preliminary Considerations

The surgeon is free to use his or her usual method of preparing and draping the patient. Anesthesia may also be delivered in the usual way, along with ocular massage. Since vitreous shrinkage is very important, intravenous mannitol or urea should be used to supplement massage. Maximal pupillary dilation may be attained with six instillations of mydriatic one to two hours prior to surgery. A moist gauze pad is placed over the patient's closed eye until the donor button has been prepared.

*Preparation of the Donor Cornea

The donor eye is removed from the storage container in the operating room. The donor eye is wrapped in sterile gauze and set on the flat surface of a sterilely draped table. An 8.5-mm trephine is placed over the corneal center. The trephine is rotated until the anterior chamber is entered in a small area. Healon is introduced into the eye until the anterior chamber is completely filled. This will help to protect the donor endothelium during button removal. Once the chamber is entered, the free edge of the donor button is grasped with a fine toothed forceps and button removal completed with corneal scissors. A mound of Healon is then placed in a small, flat sterile dish or open container, and the donor button is immersed in the mound, endothelial side facing up (Figs. 1, 2, and 3).

Trephination of Patient's Cornea

Attention is now directed to the patient's eye. The moist gauze pad is removed, and a lid speculum is placed in the eye. A muscle hook is run along the upper and lower fornices to make sure that no pressure is

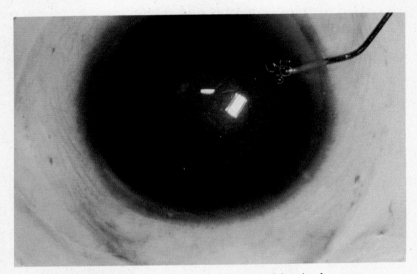

Figure 1. Injection of Healon into stab incision in donor eye.

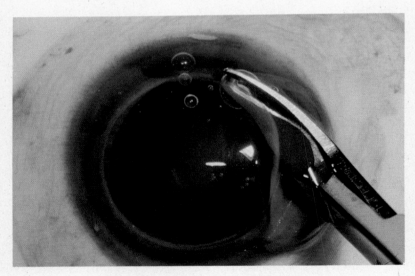

Figure 2. Cutting out donor button.

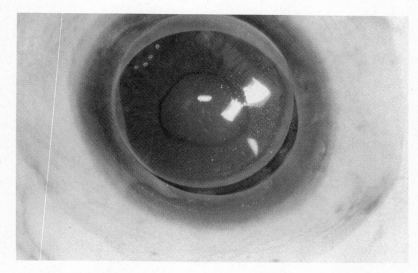

Figure 3. Donor button lying on mound of Healon in donor eye.

exerted from the speculum to the globe. An 8.5-mm trephine is adjusted onto the corneal center and rotated so as to just enter the anterior chamber in one small location. Fixation of the globe during trephination is accomplished with tissue forceps applied on the scleral side of the limbus. Once the chamber is entered, excision of the pathologic corneal button is done with a fine corneal scissors held perpendicular to the

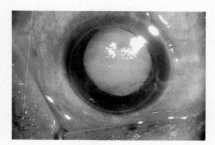

Figure 4. Picture of eye with keratoconus, cataract, and trephine groove.

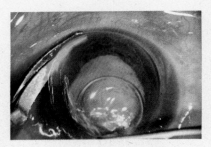

Figure 5. Scissoring out recipient cornea.

corneal surface. Any residual shelf or strand should be dissected from the sides of the opening so that the walls are relatively straight and ready to appose the sides of the donor button (Figs. 4 and 5).

*Peripheral Iridectomy

The tip of a fine, nontoothed forceps is now gently slid under the superior lip of the trephine opening and allowed to grasp the iris peripheral. A small tent of iris is pulled out of the opening and cut. The excised iris should be spread over the drape and the presence of pigment verified. If no pigment is present, the iridectomy is not complete. The remaining iris pigment epithelium may be pulled out with a nontoothed forceps.

*Extracapsular Extraction

A sharp cystotome or bent 27-gauge needle is now applied to the anterior lens capsule just central to the dilated pupillary margin and about 16 radial cuts following the pupil are made. Anterior capsulotomy may also be accomplished with fine scissors. The capsule fragment is then grasped and removed with fine forceps. The nucleus is now scooped from the capsule with a lens loop and gently lifted from the anterior chamber.

A modern irrigation–aspiration 19-gauge cannula with a 3.0-mm aspiration side port is attached to a 10-cc syringe filled with balanced salt solution and is used to remove the remaining cortex in a push/pull fashion. The small port allows selective aspiration of cortical remnants.

Irrigating Healon behind the anterior capsule, peripherally, helps float

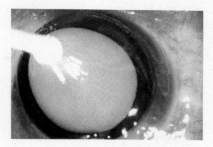

Figure 6. Cryoextraction of cataract.

the capsule forward allowing peripheral cortical remnants to be captured by the aspiration maneuver. The lens cortex mixes easily with the Healon, almost drawing the pieces of lens into the viscoelastic matrix.

As a last step, a sandblasted flat cannula is used to gently and meticulously scrape off the final material from the posterior capsule. If it is felt that the posterior capsule out to the periphery is clean, no posterior capsulotomy is necessary.

Intracapsular Cataract Extraction

For the intracapsular surgeon, this portion of the procedure is easy. The cataract is simply extracted using a cryoextractor. Zonulysis may be enzymatic or mechanical (Fig. 6).

*Posterior Lens Implantation

The lens, coated with Healon, is picked up with a smooth forceps (such as the McPherson-Kelman forceps) by grasping the lens optic itself, and the inferior loop is directed under the inferior iris and into the inferior capsular bag. The lens is then released. The open or superior end of the loop is now grasped with the forceps. With the other hand, the surgeon uses a spatula as a guide while the superior loop is compressed until it will just fit under the superior pupillary margin and slide under the superior iris. Once posterior to the iris, the loop is released and allowed to spring back to its normal size and guided to the capsule periphery. Final centration can now be accomplished with a fine hook or spatula.

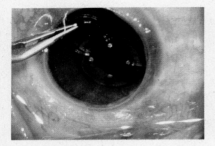

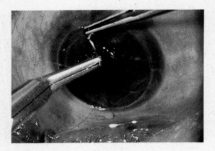

Figure 7. Lens implantation.

Figure 8. Suturing of graft, lying on bed of Healon.

Pupillary Plane Lens Implantation

The lens, coated with Healon, is picked up with a smooth forceps by grasping the anterior superior haptic and the optic itself. The inferior loops are directed toward 6 o'clock and engage the inferior iris. The lens is then pushed toward 6 o'clock, stretching the iris inferiorly until the superior loops straddle the superior iris. The forceps are then withdrawn (Fig. 7).

*Anterior Chamber Filling

The anterior chamber is now filled with Healon. About 0.5 cc is used for this purpose.

*Placement and Fixation of Donor Button

The donor button, covered with Healon, is gently grasped, avoiding endothelial touch, and fitted into the trephined opening and allowed to settle onto the bed of Healon. Using 10-0 monofilament nylon, four fixation sutures (cardinal sutures) are placed in an interrupted fashion in the four corneal quadrants. A running suture averaging six bites per quadrant and of $^1/_2$ to $^3/_4$ corneal thickness is then completed. If the chamber should start to shallow during suturing, additional Healon is pumped in. The tension of the suture is then adjusted so that wound apposition is as uniform as possible for 360°. A triple throw knot then

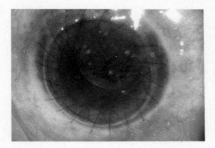

Figure 9. Sutures in place.

unites the two loose ends of the running suture. Two single throws then make the knot permanent.

At this point, some of the Healon may be removed from the anterior chamber to avoid the possible elevation of intraocular pressure during the postoperative period. For best results, gently introduce a 30-gauge cannula into the anterior chamber (between two sutures) and inject a small amount of balanced saline solution at the limbus. This maneuver should force some Healon out of the eye on the other side of the eye (Figs. 8 and 9).

Final Medication

At the close of the procedure, corticosteroids should be injected sub-conjunctivally along with an antibiotic. During the postoperative period, corticosteroid drops should be prescribed until inflammation has subsided.

REFERENCES

1. Katzin, H.M. Combined surgery for corneal transplantation and cataract extraction. *Am. J. Ophthalmol.* 62:556, 1966.
2. Casey, T.A. The combined operation of cataract and corneal graft. *Trans. Ophthalmol. Soc. U.K.* 89:659, 1969.
3. Kaufman, H.E. Combined graft and cataract extraction, in Welsh, R. (ed): *Cataract Surgery.* Miami: Educational Press 1969, p. 192.
4. Taylor, D.M. Keratoplasty and intraocular lenses. *Ophthalmic Surg.* 7:31, 1976.

5. Lee, J.R., Dohlman, C.H. Intraocular lens implantation in combination with kerato-plasty. *Ann. Ophthalmol.* 9:513, 1977.

6. Aquavella, J.V., Shaw, E.L., Rao, G.N. Intraocular lens implantation combined with penetrating keratoplasty. *Ophthalmic Surg.* 8:113, 1977.

7. Alpar, J.J. Keratoplasty and primary and secondary lens implantations. *Ophthalmic Surg.* 9:59, 1978.

8. Hunkeler, J.D., Hyde, L.L. The triple procedure: Combined penetrating keratoplasty, cataract extraction and lens implantation. *Am. Intraocular Implant Soc. J.* 5:222, 1979.

9. Lindstrom, R.L., Harris, W.S., Doughman, D.J. Combined penetrating keratoplasty, extracapsular extraction and posterior chamber lens implantation. *Am. Intraocular Implant Soc. J.* 7:130, 1981.

12
Peripheral Iridectomy Using Healon

Robert Stegmann

David Miller

Introduction

In his brief but brilliant career (he died at 42 of tuberculosis), Albrecht von Graefe gave much to ophthalmology. One of his most important contributions was the operation of broad iridectomy for acute glaucoma (1), reported in 1857. Unfortunately, the distinction between narrow angle glaucoma and open angle glaucoma was not appreciated at that time, and so von Graefe's operation did not always help the patient. In fact, he admitted that complete success after surgery was the exception rather than the rule. In 1920, Curran started to penetrate the mystery dividing the various types of glaucoma. He realized that certain forms of narrow angle glaucoma were due to pupillary block. He treated these cases with a peripheral iridotomy and reported some dramatic successes (2,3). Unhappily, Curran's operation did not work well in chronic angle closure glaucoma, where peripheral anterior synechiae had over-grown the angle. Thus, the operation lost popularity. Actually, a classification of glaucoma based on anterior chamber depth had been suggested by Raeder in 1923 (4). However, this concept received little attention until 1938, when Otto Barkan was able to incorporate all important observations that had come before by employing the gonioscopic appearance of the angle (5). He was able to then appreciate that narrow angle glaucoma produced an elevated intraocular pressure because the iris covered the trabecular meshwork. In open angle glaucoma, he suggested that the obstruction to outflow was within the trabecular meshwork. By the early 1950s, the terrain of angle closure glaucoma was in much sharper focus. Haas and Scheie (6) realized that peripheral iridectomy would only be successful if performed soon after the first attack. Finally, Paul Chandler (6) brought together the ideas and observations of the past 100 years into one clear and crisp picture of the cause, diagnosis, and treatment of angle closure glaucoma. Ultimately, Lowe applied Koch's postulates to acute angle closure glaucoma when he demonstrated the value of prophylactic peripheral iridectomy in preventing the acute attack (7,8). Today, the operation is still performed as Chandler described it in 1952. At that time, he described two important considerations during the surgery that could effect the overall outcome. First, he noted that injury to the lens or the response of the eye to surgery could produce a cataract. This observation was supported and quantitated by Godel and Regenbogen (9). He also observed that if early synechiae had formed prior to the time of surgery, the iridectomy alone might not cure the glaucoma. Thus, he advocated chamber deepening and synechia lysis at surgery. This observation was later confirmed by Playfair and Watson (10), who performed 81 peripheral iridectomies less than a week after an attack of acute angle closure glaucoma. Their long-term follow-up revealed that the operation controlled the glaucoma in 72% of the eyes. One of the primary causes of surgical failure was the presence of anterior synechiae.

It is in the prevention of these surgical failures that Healon may play a role. We have noted that after peripheral iridectomy, the chamber may be deepened with Healon, and the freshly formed synechiae can be teased apart by the gentle jet of Healon. What follows is a step-by-step description of a peripheral iridectomy. The headings preceded by an asterisk describe the way that Healon can be used to improve the results of the operation.

PERIPHERAL IRIDECTOMY

Preliminary Considerations

The surgeon may use his or her usual method of preparation and draping of the patient as well as the accustomed mode of anesthesia, along with the preferred lid speculum and superior rectus stay suture placement.

*Incision

The preferred site is at 10:30 or 1:30, so that if a filtering operation is necessary at a later date, the 12 o'clock position will be undisturbed.

Although the initiating flap may be limbus based, the fornix-based flap has the advantage of allowing an unobstructed view of the structures of the superior limbus. Thus, the conjunctiva is picked up with a pair of toothless forceps and tented. A blunt-tipped scissor is then used to make a 6–7 mm peritomy starting at the junction of cornea and conjunctiva. The conjunctiva is then dissected posteriorly for about 3–4 mm.

Because these eyes have shallow anterior chambers with an anterior position of the ciliary body, care must be taken not to catch the iris or ciliary body or injure the lens during the incision into the eye. A rounded tip blade is probably the safest blade to use. The handle of the scalpel is held nearly perpendicular to the sclera and applied 1 mm posterior to the limbus. The surgeon then makes a $^2/_3$ thickness groove into the limbus about 3–4 mm in length. In order to enter the chamber without cutting into the iris, the rest of the incision is made slowly and cautiously. An aid for the beginning surgeon is to place a suture, the depth of the groove, on either side of the incision. The assistant can now pull the wound apart, allowing the surgeon to slowly dissect into the chamber. At that moment the iris will usually prolapse into the incision without chamber loss because the pupillary block mechanism is responsible for the attack of glaucoma.

A drop or two of Healon placed on either side of the incision will lubricate the sides and allow replacement of iris after the iridectomy. If the iris does not prolapse spontaneously, gentle pressure on the posterior lip of the incision often allows the iris to pop out. If there are peripheral anterior synechiae at the site of the operation, the iris will not prolapse. To separate the synechia, the tip of a spatula is introduced into the chamber until the tip is seen. The tip of the spatula is then swept from one side to the other, lysing any adjacent synechiae present. The spatula is then withdrawn rapidly so as not to lose aqueous. If the posterior lip of the incision is now depressed, the iris should prolapse. If the iris will still not prolapse, a fine forceps with roughened apposing surfaces is used to reach into the incision and pull out a small knuckle of iris without injuring the lens. The apex of the iris knuckle is then snipped with fine scissors. The excised iris should be spread out on the drape and inspected to make sure that iris pigment is present. If none is present, additional iris with the pigment must be taken.

After the iridectomy is completed, the iris is usually caught in the incision site. By stroking the peripheral cornea first toward the corneal center and then away from the center, the iris will usually retract back into the anterior chamber.

If the prolapsed iris will still not return to the chamber, Healon may be introduced through a fine cannula into the wound anterior to the

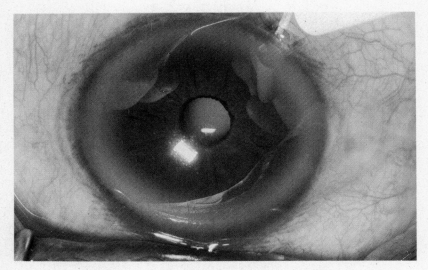

Figure 1. A scratch incision into the limbus.

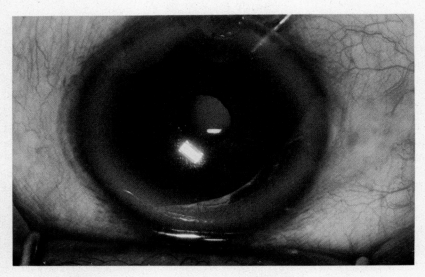

Figure 2. Deepening of anterior chamber with Healon.

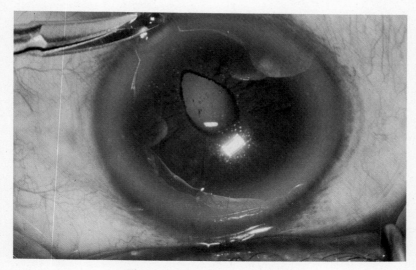

Figure 3. Excision of iris tissue.

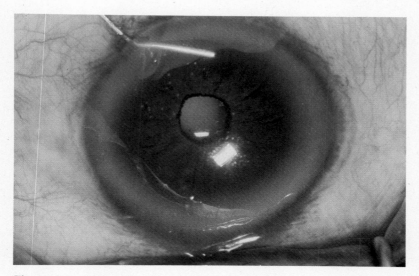

Figure 4. Breaking of synnechiae using gentle jets of Healon superiorly.

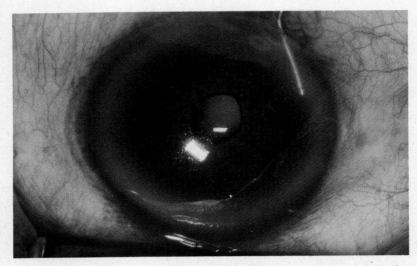

Figure 5. Breaking of synnechiae using gentle jets of Healon inferiorly.

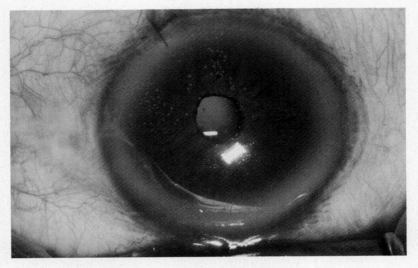

Figure 6. Closure of limbal incision.

iris. The Healon will deepen the chamber by pushing iris and lens back, and thus the prolapsed iris will be drawn into the chamber. Once the iris is properly in place, the pupil becomes round and the iridectomy is easily seen. The introduction of Healon at this time will also serve a second purpose. By deepening the chamber and pushing the iris-lens diaphragm into a slightly concave configuration, newly formed peripheral anterior synechiae will be lysed. Most of the Healon should then be gently washed from the chamber (Figs. 1–6).

Wound Closure

Usually one 8-0 catgut suture will bring the limbal wound edges together. If the wound is large, a second interrupted suture may be used.

Postoperative Care

An eye pad is placed over the closed eye and taped in place. Postoperatively, 10% phenylephrine is used twice daily for about a week along with antibiotic and steroid eye drops. The medication is stopped when the inflammation has subsided.

REFERENCES

1. Adler, F.H. Iridectomy in glaucoma (abridged translation of von Graefe's article) *Arch. Ophthalmol.* 1:71, 1929.

2. Curran, E.J. New operation for glaucoma involving a new principle in the etiology and treatment of chronic primary glaucoma. *Arch. Ophthalmol.* 49:131, 1920.

3. Curran, E.J. Peripheral irirotomy in acute and chronic glaucoma. Some results after ten years' duration. Anatomic classification of glaucoma. *Trans. Ophthalmol. Soc. U.K.* 51:520, 1931.

4. Raeder, J.G. I. Untersuchungen über die Lage und Dicke der Linse in menschlichen Augen bei physiologischen und pathologischen Zustanden nach einer neuen Gemessen. II. Die Lage der Linse bei glaukomatosen Zustanden. *Von Graefe Arch. Ophth.* 112:1, 29, 1923.

5. Barkan, O. Glaucoma: Classification, causes and surgical control. *Am. J. Ophthalmol.* 21:1099, 1938.

6. Chandler, P.A. Narrow angle glaucoma. *Arch. Ophthalmol.* 47:695, 1952.

7. Lowe, R.F. Acute angle closure glaucoma. The second eye: An analysis of 200 cases. *Br. J. Ophthalmol.* 46:641, 1962.

8. Lowe, R.F. Primary angle closure glaucoma. A review five years after bilateral surgery. *Br. J. Ophthalmol.* 57:457, 1973.

9. Godel, V., Regenbogen, L. Cataragenic factors in patients with primary angle closure glaucoma after peripheral iridectomy. *Am. J. Ophthalmol.* 83:180, 1977.

10. Playfair, T.J., Watson, P.G. Management of acute primary angle closure glaucoma: A long-term follow-up of the results of peripheral iridectomy used as an initial procedure. *Br. J. Ophthalmol.* 63:17, 1979.

13
Thermal Sclerotomy Using Healon

Robert Stegmann

David Miller

Introduction

Albrecht von Graefe must also be considered the father of filtration surgery for glaucoma control. Ironically, however, he considered the filtering bleb that resulted from over 20% of his iridectomies to be an example of undesirable healing rather than the real reason that the operation succeeded (1). He thought that the removal of iris tissue was the principal pressure lowering mechanism of the operation. Of course, his misconception was understandable. The distinction between narrow angle glaucoma and open angle glaucoma was not appreciated at that time. Thus, his iridectomy worked in cases of acute narrow angle glaucoma, and his iridectomy followed by anomalous healing with a cystoid cicatrix worked in cases of open angle glaucoma. However, his iridectomy followed by the formation of a tight scar at the incision site failed in the cases of open angle glaucoma and in most cases of chronic narrow angle glaucoma. As you might expect, von Graefe's strong advocacy of an operation that had only a modest record of success attracted strong criticism, again not always for the right reasons. In 1858, an article by Jones and MacKenzie (2) advocated paracentesis and stated, "Iridectomy opposed the plainest principles of surgery and common sense." The authors went on to state that they had no doubt that in a short time iridectomy would be abandoned in favor of frequent paracenteses. Von Graefe responded to this strongly worded article in a paper (3) in which he stated that, in his experience, paracentesis did not work. He then closed with one of the most dignified "put downs" in the history of ophthalmology. "I willingly pardon older and so highly deserving men for their want of that elasticity requisite for the immediate reception of new views, but I should have indeed expected more moderation from the Nestor of English Ophthalmology."

Interestingly, von Graefe's iridectomy remained the most commonly used operation for glaucoma control on the continent until the turn of the century. However, resistance was mounting. At the Ophthalmological Society Meeting in Heidelberg in both 1869 and 1871, Louis Wecker (4) (later to be ennobled Louis de Wecker) voiced the opinion that it was not the excision of iris tissue but the incision of sclera that embodied von Graefe's glaucoma operation. He reasoned that the pressure lowering effect of the surgery was due to the imperfect apposition of the wound lips resulting in a filtering cicatrix. De Wecker's own technique of producing a scleral flap resembled portions of modern-day trabeculectomy. By the early 1900s, support grew stronger for the principle of a filtering sclerotomy. However, opinions differed as to the most effective method. LaGrange recommended excision of the anterior lip of the scleral incision (5). Holth (6) invented a punch that automatically cut out a semielliptical piece of one side of the posterior scleral lip. Elliot, in an effort to make a precise excision of sclera in the inflamed eyes that he was working on in India, developed a series of small trephines (7). The Elliot operation remained the most popular antiglaucoma operation for many years (8) until the thermal sclerotomy was introduced almost concurrently by Preziosi (9) and Scheie (10). The latter reported a relatively short-term percentage rate of success in the 1980s, which has since been confirmed by others (11). However, over a longer period, Mishima projects the probability of success to be about 50% (personal communication, 1981). The simple, deliberate scleral incision followed by thermal cautery to the wound edges was technically easier to perform than the Elliot trephination in cases of shallow anterior chamber and narrow entrance to the chamber angle. Since the scleral incision can be done under precise visual control, the operation also produces a lower incidence of accidental penetration of the lens or the ciliary body. However, thermal sclerotomy also has complications. The formation of postoperative anterior synechias will eliminate a meager trabecular meshwork outflow channel that could be useful if the filtration fistula should close. Thus, eventual closure of the filtration fistula becomes a related complication. A second major complication of filtration surgery is the postoperative development of a cataract. This complication is usually caused by lens trauma at the time of the surgery. Chandler and Grant (12) suggest that the two principal causes of the postoperative flat chamber are decreased rate of aqueous formation and excessive aqueous runoff through the scleral opening. They feel that if the eye is soft postoperatively, a separation of ciliary body and/or choroid results and aqueous formation declines.

Healon seems to play an important role in preventing this complication. A deeply formed, Healon-filled chamber should produce a slower egress of aqueous out of the trabecular meshwork and scleral incision than a saline- or air-filled chamber. A full chamber and a firmer eye should theoretically decrease the chances of ciliary body separation and thus maintain a more normal secretion of aqueous. By filling the bleb with Healon at the close of surgery, a tamponade effect should result in a slower runoff of aqueous into a bleb in the early postoperative period. Therefore, the use of Healon should lower the incidence of postoperative flat chamber after filtering surgery. Our experience to date seems to bear out this contention that Healon may lower but not eliminate the incidence of postoperative flat chamber.

Good bleb filtration requires thin succulent conjunctival tissue. To maintain conjunctiva in such a state, there must be minimal conjunctival drying and trauma during the surgery. Healon can play an important role toward this end. Retracted conjunctival tissue can be immersed in Healon to prevent drying. Healon can also be used to dissect the conjunctiva early in the surgery. These steps should minimize postoperative conjunctival fibrosis.

In the pages to follow, a step-by-step description of a thermal sclerotomy combined with an iridectomy will be described. The headings preceded by an asterisk describe the way that Healon can be used to improve the results of the operation.

THERMAL SCLEROTOMY AND IRIDECTOMY

Preliminary Considerations

The surgeon may use his or her usual method of preparation and draping of the patient as well as the accustomed mode of anesthesia and placement of the surgeon's favorite lid speculum.

Superior Rectus Suture

In order to give the surgeon ample superior conjunctiva to work with, the superior rectus suture should be placed more posterior than usual. To achieve this posterior position, the assistant rotates the globe downward maximally. The surgeon grasps the conjunctiva 10–12 mm above the limbus with a toothless forceps and pulls it downward toward the limbus, almost heaping redundant conjunctiva onto the limbus. The surgeon then grasps the superior rectus with a toothed forceps (behind the first forceps). The first forceps is then released and the fixation suture inserted.

Conjunctival Flap

Conjunctiva and Tenon's capsule are then pierced with a scissors just anterior to the superior rectus suture and about a 5 mm incision is made around the 12 o'clock position. The flap is now bluntly dissected down to the limbus. Chandler and Grant (12) suggest the limbal incision be at 11 or 1 o'clock so that if a second operation is required, there is room to do it in the same region (Fig. 1).

Scleral Incision

Mild cautery is circumferentially applied to the line of the future limbal incision for 3–5 mm. Holding a rounded blade almost perpendicular to the iris, the surgeon now makes a groove of half thickness along the

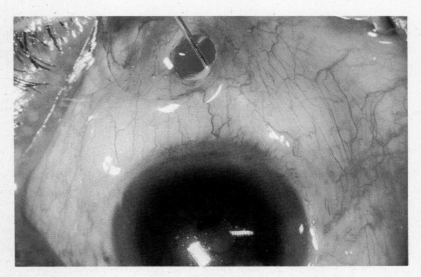

Figure 1. Dissection of conjunctiva and Tenon's capsule down to limbus using Healon.

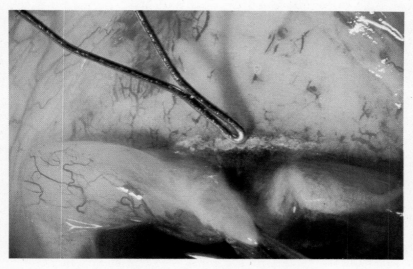

Figure 2. Marking groove at limbus with cautery.

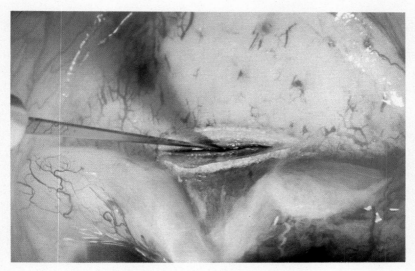

Figure 3. Cutting into cauterized groove with blade.

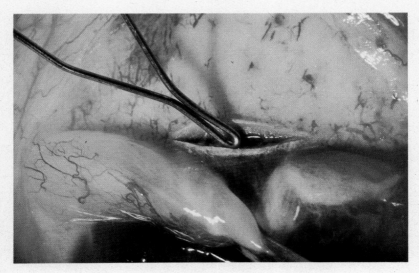

Figure 4. Use of cautery to enlarge incision.

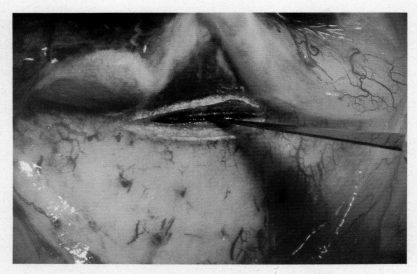

Figure 5. Entering anterior chamber with blade.

previously cauterized area. Very light cautery is then reapplied along the side of the groove, retracting, but not charring the groove. All bleeders in the area should also be gently closed with cautery. The limbal incision is deepened with a rounded blade and cautery reapplied. Entrance into the chamber is announced by a puff of aqueous. The incision is enlarged to 5 mm with the knife blade. Because of the cautery-induced shrinkage, the incision should be almost sausage-shaped and measure 1 mm by 5 mm (Figs. 2, 3, 4, and 5).

Iridectomy

If there are no synechiae in the area, the iris should prolapse through the newly made opening. If the iris does not prolapse spontaneously, a fine spatula is introduced into the incision, anterior to the iris, and swept from side to side so as to lyse adjacent synechiae. Now gentle pressure on the posterior scleral lip should induce the iris to prolapse. The iris root is grasped with forceps, tented up gently, and excised. The excised iris should then be spread along the drape and inspected for iris pigment. If no pigment is present, the iridectomy must be completed (Figs. 6 and 7).

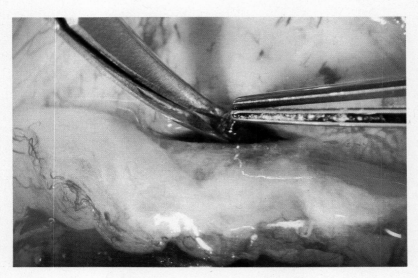

Figure 6. Performing the iridectomy.

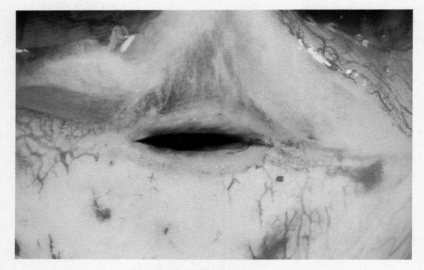

Figure 7. Iridectomy complete.

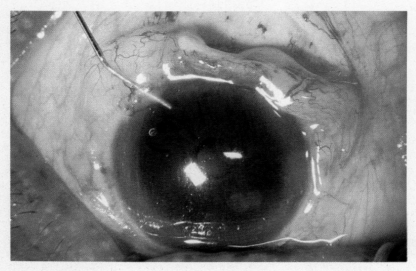

Figure 8. Filling anterior chamber with Healon through scratch incision.

*Restoration of the Anterior Chamber

Using a cannula attached to a Healon syringe, the iris pillars are repositioned in the anterior chamber by a gentle jet of Healon. Care must be taken not to touch the lens with the cannula tip. The anterior chamber is now deepened with Healon until the iris-lens diaphragm takes on a flat configuration (Fig. 8).

Wound Closure

Closure of Tenon's capsule is accomplished with a running absorbable suture. Overlying conjunctiva is now sutured closed with a similar suture.

*Bleb Priming

A sharp 27 needle is attached to the Healon syringe, and small amounts of Healon are injected under the future bleb site. Healon is also injected under conjunctiva all around the limbus producing a donut-ring appearance. Experience has shown that this maneuver encourages a diffuse flat bleb (Figs. 9 and 10).

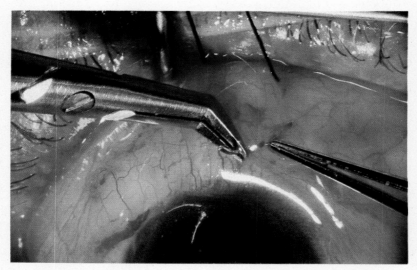

Figure 9. Closing conjunctiva and Tenon's capsule, layer by layer.

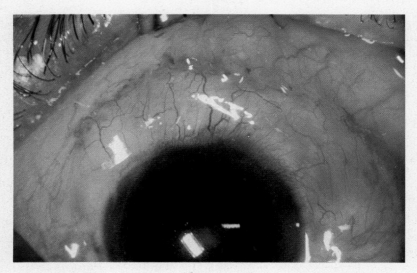

Figure 10. Ballooning of subconjunctival space with Healon.

Postoperative Medication

Subconjunctival injection of a corticosteroid is recommended in the 6 o'clock position at the close of surgery. Corticosteroid drops should then be administered (three times a day) for the first few postoperative weeks.

REFERENCES

1. Von Graefe, A. Weitere Zusätze über Glaukom und die Heilwirkung der Iridectomie. *Arch. Ophthalmol.* 8:243, 1861.

2. Jones, T.W., MacKenzie, W. Operation of iridectomy or excision of piece of iris. *Med. Times and Gazette* 16:342, 1858.

3. Von Graefe, A. On iridectomy, in iritis, iridochoroiditis, and glaucoma. *Med. Times and Gazette* 16:447, 1858.

4. De Wecker, L. Die Sklerotomie als Glaukom Operation. *Ber. Ophth. Ges.* 8:305, 1871.

5. LaGrange, F. De l'iridectomie et de la sclerectomie combinees dans le traitement du glaucoma chronique. Procéde nouveau pour l'établissement de la cicatrice filtrante. *Bull. Mem. Soc. Fr. Ophtalmol.* 23:477, 1906.

6. Holth, S. A new technique in punch forceps sclerectomy for chronic glaucoma. *Br. J. Ophthalmol.* 5:544, 1921.

7. Elliot, R.H. A preliminary note on a new operative procedure for the establishment of a filtering cicatrix in the treatment of glaucoma. *Ophthalmoscope* 7:804, 1909.

8. Sugar, H.S. The filtering operations: An historical review. *Glaucoma* 3:85, 1981.

9. Preziosi, L. The flap and filtration in Presiosi's: Operation for glaucoma. *Trans. Ophthalmol. Soc. U.K.* 57:675, 1957.

10. Scheie, H.G. Retraction of scleral wound edges as a fistulizing procedure for glaucoma. *Am. J. Ophthalmol.* 45:220, 1958.

11. Drance, S.M., Vargass, E. Trabeculectomy and thermosclerectomy: A comparison of two procedures. *Can. J. Ophthalmol.* 8:413, 1973.

12. Chandler, P.A., Grant, W.M. *Lectures in Glaucoma.* Philadelphia, Lea & Febiger, 1972.

14
Trabeculectomy Using Healon

Robert Stegman

David Miller

Introduction

Although the filtering sclerotomy operation has succeeded in many patients, it is not without complications and failure. The high incidence of postoperative flat chambers (up to 45%) (1), cataract formation (up to 36%) (2), and the frightening appearance of late endophthalmitis in patients with thin cystic blebs (2) all seemed to call for a better operation. Certainly, any operation that simply made a hole in the eye was not in keeping with the sophisticated science of the 1960s. A lead for a new approach came from the basic studies of Goldmann (3,4) and Grant (5), who demonstrated that the site of the lesion in open angle glaucoma was in the outflow channels. In 1958, Grant (6) removed the trabecular meshwork of an enucleated eye and showed a marked increase in aqueous outflow. This finding, along with the increased appreciation for surgery under the microscope, set the stage for the surgical innovator. In 1960, Redmond Smith reported success with an operation in which he threaded a nylon filament in through Schlemm's canal and used it to rip an opening into the trabecular meshwork (7). In the same year, Krasnov reported good results when he exteriorized Schlemm's canal and opened its outer wall (8). The trend continued to excise the diseased tissue in the glaucoma patient. Thus, excision of a portion of the trabecular meshwork seemed a logical next step. Sugar tried it first and reported failure (9). However, Coryllos (10) and Cairns (11) tried it and reported success. Both felt that they were removing damaged tissue and allowing drainage into the open ends of Schlemm's canal. However, with time it became clear that trabeculectomy worked because it filtered aqueous around the scleral flap. In a sense the debate as to how the operation worked was reminiscent of the debate over how von Graefe's broad iridectomy worked. But whereas the debate over iridectomy raged for almost 50 years before it was agreed the sclerotomy filtration was the mechanism of success, the trabeculectomy issue was concluded in five years. First, Spencer (12) showed histologically that filtration into the cut ends of Schlemm's canal would be unlikely because the cut ends were fibrosed closed. Then, many surgeons noted that most patients with a lowered pressure did have filtering blebs (13,14). Finally, histologic examination of the excised tissue from successful surgical cases revealed that very often tissue other than the trabecular meshwork was removed (2). Thus, in the end, trabeculectomy was seen as an operation with a short-term success rate of over 90% that worked via a scleral filtration mechanism (15,16,17). It should be noted that Mishima projects the probability of long-term success to be 50% (personal communication, 1981). It was also seen as an operation that was capable of lowering intraocular pressure to about 18 mm Hg (18,19). Therefore, if optic nerve damage dictates the necessity of achieving lower levels of pressure, then the older forms of filtering are suggested (20).

Unhappily, trabeculectomy is not without complications and problems. Flat chambers, cataracts, and uveitis can occur postoperatively, and a significant number of patients must supplement the operative results with medication (2,20,21).

It would appear that Healon may help to reduce the number of such complications. Pape and Balazs (22) reported only one postoperative flat chamber after 15 trabeculectomies using Healon. However, we must admit that we have seen flat chambers after performing trabeculectomy with Healon.

Good bleb filtration requires thin succulent conjunctival tissue. To maintain conjunctiva in such a state, there must be minimal conjunctival drying and trauma during the surgery. Healon can play an important role toward this end. Retracted conjunctival tissue can be immersed in Healon to prevent drying. Healon can also be used to dissect the conjunctiva early in the surgery. These steps should minimize postoperative conjunctival fibrosis. Our experience does confirm the fact that the blebs are more succulent after Healon usage.

A step-by-step description of a trabeculectomy will follow. The headings preceded by an asterisk describe the way that Healon can be used to improve the results of the operation.

TRABECULECTOMY

Preliminary Considerations

The surgeon may use his or her usual method of preparation and draping of the patient as well as the accustomed mode of anesthesia, along with the preferred lid speculum and bridle suture.

*Conjunctival-Fascial Flap

About 2 cc of anesthetic are introduced below Tenon's capsule, just anterior to the bridle suture, to balloon Tenon's fascia and conjunctiva. An incision is made, anterior to the bridle suture, with blunt scissors through both layers to bare sclera. The incision should extend between 10 to 2 o'clock. The flap can be dissected forward with the spreading of the blunt scissors or by using a moistened tightly wound cotton tipped applicator. Care must be taken to close all bleeders during the dissection. The dissection is continued to the limbus. The retracted conjunctival tissue should be covered by Healon to prevent tissue drying and enhanced postoperative inflammation (Figs. 1 and 2).

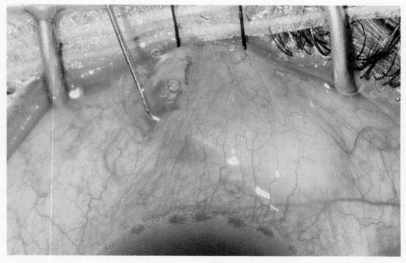

Figure 1. Ballooning up of conjunctiva and Tenon's capsule with Healon.

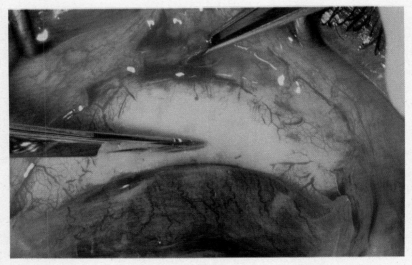

Figure 2. Dissection of conjunctiva and Tenon's capsule down to the limbus.

Trabeculectomy

The flap is rolled onto the cornea, exposing the superior limbus. Calipers are used to measure and mark a 4 × 4 mm square scleral trapdoor hinged at the limbus (meeting of white and blue zone). The scleral flap of $^1/_2$–$^2/_3$ scleral thickness is then developed by using either a razor blade knife or rounded blade. The flap is now retracted onto the cornea. Along the hinge of the flap, a 1.5 × 4 mm strip of remaining sclera with underlying scleral spur and trabecular meshwork is now dissected away. The dissection may be started with a razor blade knife and completed elevating the flap with a fine toothed forceps and cutting out the flap with a fine scissors.

At this stage, a knuckle of iris will usually prolapse through the new opening. This iris is grasped and an iridectomy is performed. The excised iris should be spread out to see if pigment epithelium is present. If none is present, the iridectomy must be completed.

The scleral flap is now returned to its original position and two 10-0 interrupted nylon sutures are tightly tied at the corners of the square. The conjunctiva is then closed with a running suture (Figs. 3–10).

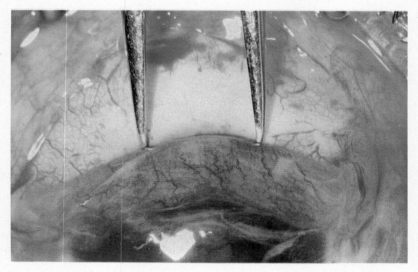

Figure 3. Marking the potential scleral flap area with calipers.

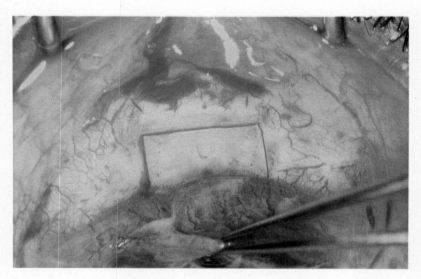

Figure 4. Marking of scleral flap with blade.

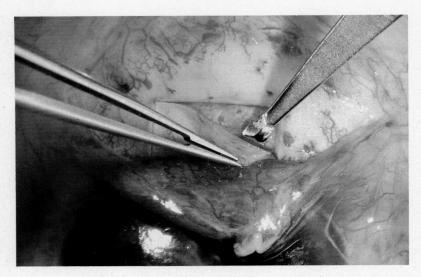

Figure 5. Dissection of the scleral flap.

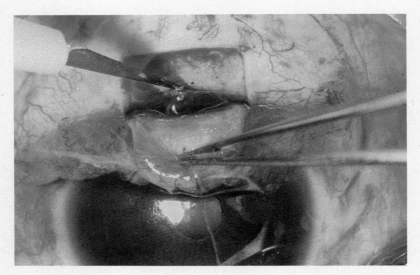

Figure 6. Dissection of window of trabecular meshwork.

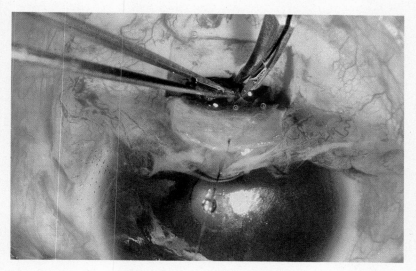

Figure 7. Peripheral iridectomy.

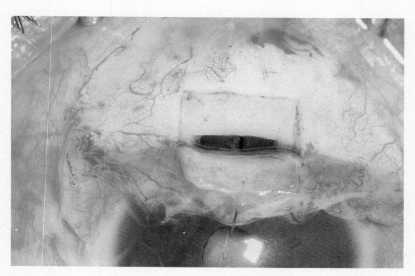

Figure 8. Appearance of operative field after peripheral iridectomy.

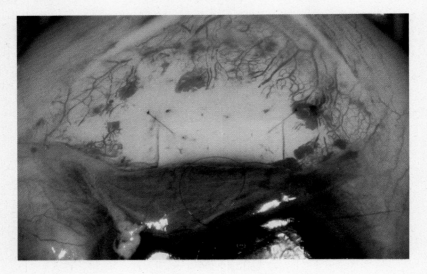

Figure 9. Scleral flap sutured in place.

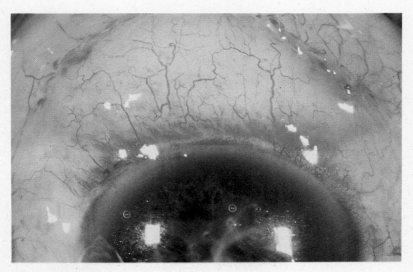

Figure 10. Appearance of eye at the end of the case with conjunctiva ballooned with Healon.

*The Role of Healon

In cases of chronic angle closure glaucoma, a stream of Healon may often break newly formed synechiae. After the iridectomy, Healon is injected into the anterior chamber. The fine cannula moves gently around the limbus, driving Healon into the angle structures, stretching and breaking synechiae wherever possible. The chamber should be deep and completely filled with Healon at the close of the procedure. Finally, Healon should be injected via a sharp 27-gauge needle into the sub-Tenon's fascia space where the filtration bleb will reside. This maneuver prepares the area for aqueous collection. The presence of Healon also prevents overrun of aqueous into the bleb area for the first few post-operative days.

REFERENCES

1. Chandler, P.A., Grant, W.M. *Lectures in Glaucoma.* Philadelphia, Lea & Febiger, 1972, p. 298.
2. Watson, P.G. Trabeculectomy, in *Controversies in Ophthalmology:* Borochoff, A., Hutchinson, T.B., Lessell, S. (eds), 1977, p. 190.
3. Goldmann, A. An analysis of primary glaucoma. *Trans. Ophthalmol. Soc. U.K.* 69:445, 1949.
4. Goldmann, H. Die Kammewassen und das Poisaeilie Sehe Gets. *Ophthalmologica* 118:496, 1945.
5. Grant, W.M. Clinical measurements of aqueous outflow. *Arch. Ophthalmol.* 46:11, 1951.
6. Grant, W.M. Further studies on facility of flow through the trabecular meshwork. *Arch. Ophthalmol.* 60:523, 1958.
7. Smith, R.J.H. A new technique for opening the canal of Schlemm. Preliminary report. *Br. J. Ophthalmol.* 44:370, 1960.
8. Krasnov, M.M. Microsurgery of glaucoma. Indications and choice of technique. *Am. J. Ophthalmol.* 67:857, 1969.
9. Sugar, H.S. Experimental trabeculectomy in glaucoma. *Am. J. Ophthalmol.* 51:623, 1961.
10. Coryllos, D. Trabeculectomy: A new glaucoma operation. *Bull. Hellenic Ophthalmol. Soc.* 35:147, 1967.
11. Cairns, J.E. Trabeculectomy. *Am. J. Ophthalmol.* 66:673, 1968.
12. Spencer, W.H. Histologic evaluation of microsurgical glaucoma. *Trans. Am. Acad. Ophthalmol and Otolaryngol.* 76:389, 1972.
13. Cairns, J.E. Microsurgery of the outflow channels: Trabeculectomy. *Trans. Am. Acad. Ophthalmol.* 76:384, 1972.
14. Schwartz, A.L., Anderson, D.R. Trabecular surgery. *Arch. Ophthalmol.* 92:134, 1974.
15. Ridgeway, A.E.A., Rubinstein, K., Smith, V.H. Trabeculectomy. *Br. J. Ophthalmol.* 56:511, 1972.

16. Watson, P.G. Trabeculectomy, a modified ab externo technique. *Ann. Ophthalmol.* 2:199, 1970.

17. Drance, S.M., Vargass, E. Trabeculectomy and thermoscleractomy: A comparison of two procedures. *Can. J. Ophthalmol.* 8:413, 1973.

18. Jay, J.L., Murray, S.B. Characteristics of reduction of intraocular pressure after trabeculectomy. *Br. J Ophthalmol.* 64:432, 1980.

19. Jerndal, T., Lundstrom, M. 330 trabeculectomies. A long time study (3–5½ years). *Acta Ophthalmol.* 58:941, 1980.

20. Spaeth, G.L. Trabeculectomy—a good operative procedure, in Brockhurst, R., Hutchinson, B.T., Lessell, S.: *In its Place in Controversies in Ophthalmology.* Philadelphia, Lea & Febiger, 1977, p.201.

21. McPherson, S.D., Jr., Cline, J.W., McCurdy, D. Recent advances in glaucoma surgery. Trabeculotomy and trabeculectomy. *Ann. Ophthalmol.* 9:91, 1977.

22. Pape, L.G., Balazs, E.A. The use of sodium hyaluronate (Healon) in human anterior segment surgery. *Ophthalmology* 87:699, 1980.

15

War-Related Ocular Surgery: Foreign Body Removal and Repair of Corneal Laceration Using Healon

Robert Stegmann

David Miller

Introduction

As one studies the hospital records of the wars of the past 100 years, a curious fact emerges. The proportion of wounds to the eye to wounds in general has risen at an incredible pace. The percent of eye injury to body injury was 0.81% in the American Civil War (1). It rose to 1.75% in the Crimean War (1), and then to over 2.5% in the Russo–Turkish War (1). By World War I it was 8% (2) and in World War II it averaged 9% (2–6). In the Korean War eye injury-related admissions amounted to 12% (7) of all admissions, and in the 1973 Arab–Israeli War the number reached 17% (8). At first, it is difficult to understand why the eyeball, which represents $1/375$ of the total body surface, should be injured so frequently in modern war. John Bellows (2) suggests that in modern war the soldier often finds himself in the protected environment of the trench, tank, or airplane cockpit. To see the events surrounding him, he must expose his head and eyes. Since bullets and shell fragments are the emissaries of injury, and a helmet protects only the head, the eyes become victim to a disproportional number of flying missiles and booby trap fragments. It might be instructive to inspect the typical spectrum of eye casualties seen during a modern war. Bellows (2) carefully reviewed 300 eye casualties in World War II and reported the following categories:

Blunt trauma (nonperforating injury)	18%
Ocular rupture (needing immediate enucleation)	35%
Penetrating injury (with foreign body)	21%
Penetrating injury (no foreign body present)	12%
Injuries to eye adnexa (lids, muscles)	10%
Burns	3%

Since the penetrating injuries require surgical repair, this category is of greatest interest to the ophthalmic surgeon. Scott and Michaelson (9) analyzed the site of entry of 76 penetrating foreign body injuries during World War II and found that 37% entered via the cornea, 33% via the limbus, 26% via the sclera, and 4% were undetermined.

The philosophy of treatment has changed drastically as the fear of sympathetic ophthalmia has diminished. During World War I, Felix LaGrange wrote (1), "We have not met with a single case of partial rupture of the sclera permitting the eye to survive and keep its appearance after injury." In light of such findings, LaGrange and the surgeons that worked with him felt that such eyes might as well be enucleated since they had the potential of causing sympathetic ophthalmia in the uninjured eye. Interestingly, LaGrange recorded five cases of sympathetic ophthalmia out of the 2,554 eye injuries he saw.

As the percentage of eye casualties has risen in modern warfare, so has the percentage of eyes that can be repaired and saved. This is in part due to a change in the style of warfare. Whereas, shell fragments accounted for twice the number of eye injuries that were produced by bullets in World War I, they outnumbered bullet-derived injuries by 5 to 1 in World War II (2). A bullet injury to the eye is more apt to dismember the entire eye, whereas the shell fragment (Stallard (10) found they averaged 2 mm × 3 mm in size) would usually produce a tear that might be repaired. Of course, there are other important reasons for the higher salvage rate of eyes in modern warfare. With time, the philosophy of treatment changed. During the time of the Vietnam War, the American ophthalmologist, Frank Hoefle, working on board the Naval hospital ship *Repose*, wrote (11), "If there was any chance of saving an eye regardless of vision, the eye was sutured. As in Korea, no cases of sympathetic ophthalmia were seen. This confirmed our policy of avoiding enucleation where possible regardless of vision and despite the risk of sympathetic ophthalmia." It is only fair to note that, although modern techniques have reduced the incidence of sympathetic ophthalmia to less than 0.2% of all traumatically penetrated eyes, the disease has not been eliminated (12).

Finally, better prognosis in eye injury has resulted from faster evacuation of the injured to well-equipped hospitals, where there are better surgical instruments used by better trained surgeons with improved surgical techniques. The microscopes, fine sutures, sharper needles, antibiotics, and anti-inflammatory agents have all made a big difference. To this armamentarium, we think that Healon should be added. Its use in treatment of ocular trauma may be its most important contribution. In contrast to the tissue disruption of a surgical incision where the wound edges are straight and easily identifiable, the wound edges produced by a flying missile are often dirty, jagged, and covered with blood. To make matters worse, these difficult wounds must be repaired in the face of a collapsed globe. By pumping Healon into such eyes, the normal spherical configuration is reinstated and the wound edges can be more leisurely inspected, debrided, and more accurately sutured together. At the close of surgery, Healon holds the ocular structures in normal relation to each other and helps prevent dangerous adhesion formation. The following chapters will not describe the surgical repair of every type of penetrating wound, but only a few common types. In this particular chapter, the repair of a corneal laceration holding the offending foreign body will be described in detail.

FOREIGN BODY REMOVAL AND REPAIR OF CORNEAL LACERATION

Preliminary Considerations

Perform as many preliminary diagnostic tests as possible to learn about the size, position, and number of foreign bodies present. Then take specimens for culture and smear from the cul-de-sac and check for both bacteria and fungi. Tetanus toxoid is then administered, along with local and systemic broad spectrum antibiotics. Recall that infective endophthalmitis is associated with about 10% of all penetrating injuries caused by magnetic intraocular foreign bodies (13). Finally, prevention of vomiting is mandatory, as vomiting can surely cause loss of intraocular contents. Thus, preoperative intramuscular injection of chlorpromazine or prochlorperazine is recommended (14).

Whenever possible, general anesthesia should be employed for cases of perforating ocular injury. However, great care must be used in placing the endotracheal tube into the patient so that the patient does not cough or gag.

If lid edema or hemorrhage is present, placement of a speculum will place unnecessary pressure on the globe. Such pressure on the globe could expel intraocular structures. Thus, lid sutures are recommended. Make three continuous bites along the length of the upper lid margin (just beyond the lash margin) using a double-armed, 4-0 silk suture. Two vertical bites are then made deep in the lid tissue going from lid margin to lid fold and including tarsal plate. Specifically, one bite is made medially with the needle of the medial end of the suture, and the other is made laterally with the other needle. The same is done for the lower lid with another double-armed suture. Traction is then applied on the nasal, lateral ends as well as medial loop of the suture to open the eye.

*Foreign Body Removal

In this particular case, the foreign body is still in the wound. Its presence has kept the wound plugged and the anterior chamber formed. Any attempt to suddenly remove the foreign body will collapse the chamber and possibly damage the lens with the back of the foreign body. To maintain the chamber during removal of the foreign body, Healon should be used. A sharp, 27- or 30-gauge needle is placed on the barrel of the Healon syringe. The needle is then introduced into the anterior chamber at the limbus with a gentle twirling action. Once the anterior chamber is entered, Healon is introduced until the chamber is deep. The needle is then withdrawn. The foreign body is then grasped and slowly removed from the entry site. The wound edges are carefully inspected for dirt, rust, and other foreign matter. Gentle debridement of the wound edges is then undertaken. If the iris is incarcerated in the wound, it should be gently teased back into the eye. After wound closure, a peripheral iridectomy should be done in the traditional manner (Figs. 1–8).

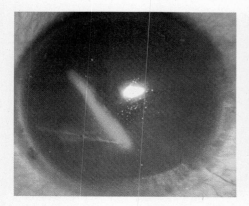

Figure 1. Preoperative appearance of the eye with foreign body in anterior chamber.

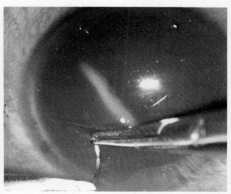

Figure 2. Placement of suture in corneal wound.

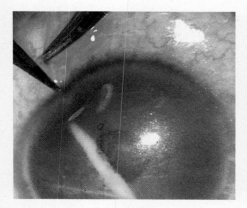

Figure 3. Stab incision at limbus.

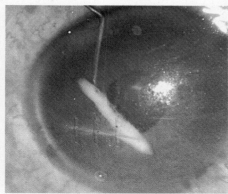

Figure 4. Introduction of Healon into the anterior chamber through a small "puncture" incision.

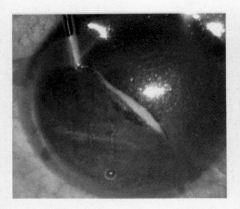

Figure 5. Grasping of foreign body with forceps (lens protected by blanket of Healon).

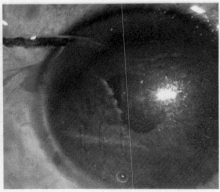

Figure 6. Removing foreign body from the eye (with loss of anterior chamber or endothelial touch).

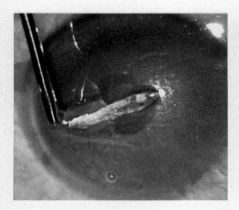

Figure 7. Size and configuration of the foreign body with respect to the eye.

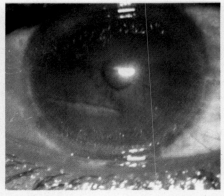

Figure 8. Appearance of eye 72 hours after surgery.

Wound Closure

A sharp reverse cutting needle on a 9-0 or 10-0 nylon suture will give the least traumatic closure. The needle bite should be at $\frac{1}{2}$ to $\frac{2}{3}$ corneal depth and about 1–2 mm from the wound edge. Care should be taken with each interrupted suture to just approximate the wound edges. It should be remembered that the wound edges will swell and make a well-approximated wound water tight.

Final Measures

At the end of the procedure, a subconjunctival injection of corticosteroids and antibiotics should be given. The dressing should include an eye pad and firm plastic or metal shield. Postoperatively, local corticosteroids and antibiotics should be continued until successful healing is assured. Use of periodic, short-acting mydriatics will help prevent posterior synechias.

REFERENCES

1. LaGrange, F. (H. Child, trans.) *Fractures of the Orbit and Injuries to the Eye in War.* London, University of London Press, 1918.
2. Bellows, J.G. Observations on 300 consecutive cases of ocular war injuries. *Am. J. Ophthalmol.* 30:309, 1947.
3. Loewenstein, A. Eye casualties at the front. *Glasgow Med. J.* 132:169, 1939.
4. MacFee, W.F. The treatment of air force combat injuries. *Ann. Surg.* 120:1, 1944.
5. Schench, H.P., Silcos, L.E., Godfrey, E.W. Eye casualties treated on a hospital ship. *U.S. Naval Med. Bull.* 42:802, 1944.
6. Wiser, H.S. Eye injuries in war casualties aboard a hospital ship. *U.S. Naval Med. Bull.* 46:67, 1946.
7. Hull, F.E. Management of eye casualties in the Far East Command during the Korean Conflict. *Trans. Am. Acad. Ophthalmol. and Otolaryngol.* 55:885, 1951.
8. Belkin, M. et al. War eye injuries with special reference to foreign bodies. *Harefuah* 91:291, 339, 403, 450, 1976.
9. Scott, G.I., Michaelson, I.C. An analysis and follow-up of 301 cases of battle casualty injury to the eye. *Br. J. Ophthalmol.* 30:42, 1946.
10. Stallard, H.B. War surgery of the eye. *Br. J. Ophthalmol.* 27:449, 1943.
11. Hoefle, F.B. Initial treatment of eye injuries. First Corps Area of Vietnam, 1966. *Arch. Ophthalmol.* 79:33, 1968.
12. Liddy, B., St.L., Stuart, J.: Sympathetic ophthalmia in Canada. *Can. J. Ophthalmol.* 7:157, 1972.
13. Michels, R.G. Vitrectomy methods in penetrating ocular trauma. *Ophthalmology* 87:629, 1980.
14. Colvin, J. Effective management of penetrating eye injuries in remote Australia. *Med. J. Aust.* 1:329, 1981.

16

Civilian-Related Ocular Injury: Repair of a Corneal Laceration Using Healon

Robert Stegmann

David Miller

Introduction

Civilian eye injuries form a significant part of the spectrum of ocular problems seen by the ophthalmologist. Actually, about 10% of all ophthalmic patients seen in a large eye clinic are there because of an eye injury (1). This percentage can climb considerably (up to 50%) in a highly industrialized city like Sheffield, England (1). Interestingly, eye injuries also comprise about 10% of all the admissions to a large, general hospital (1). Of the eye injured population, children under 14 years of age account for between 15 to 20% of all serious eye injuries. Yet, if you eliminate industrial accidents from the statistics, children are the victims of almost 50% of all eye injuries (1). A review of the types of serious eye injuries seen in adults reveals that about 15% are of the perforating variety, whereas in children about 40% of the serious eye injuries are perforating in nature (1). The prognosis of perforating injuries is often measured in terms of the percentage of eyes that ultimately must be enucleated. By the late 1960s, the enucleation rate for perforating in-

juries in adults was in the order of 15-20% (1). In children the enucleation rate for perforating injuries was almost double that figure. Although
all these figures suggest the extreme seriousness of an eye injury, they
do not reflect the progress that has been made within the twentieth
century in improving the outcome.

The greatest improvement in prognosis has occurred with anterior
segment lacerations. Up until 1945, 38% of adult eyes sustaining corneal
or corneoscleral lacerations were reported lost, and many others had
significant loss of useful vision. However, within recent years only 17%
of 419 eyes with corneal or corneoscleral lacerations were lost in two
representative series (2–5). In fact, Eagling (2) noted a final visual acuity
of 20/40 or better in 87% of cases with corneal or corneal and lens
damage by penetrating injury. Unhappily, the outlook for severe injuries
involving the posterior segment associated with significant vitreous loss
continues to be poor.

It is even worse if damaged lens tissue mixes with vitreous. Between
40 and 70% of these eyes are lost (6–8), and an average of only 13%
achieve vision of 20/40 or better (2,8). A review of these statistics can
suggest some surprising conclusions. The eye, a very specialized organ
with each element responsible for a very precise function, does not appear to possess the regenerative capacity seen in liver or bone, nor even
the healing capability of skin. In fact, if left without the help of surgical
repair, most corneal lacerations heal badly (retrocorneal membranes,
epithelial fistulas, synechia, etc.). Happily, as surgical and medical technology has improved, healing has become more controlled and visual
prognosis has become better. However, even with the help of sophisticated surgery, anterior segment injuries are still subject to the development of synechia, corneal vascularization, and astigmatism, which prevent a perfect outcome.

It would appear that the eye's limited healing ability can be mobilized
to repair most small anterior segment perforations, although imper-
fectly. Modern surgical techniques then control and direct this primitive
repair capacity to a favorable outcome in most cases. Unhappily, the
picture can change considerably if the lens is damaged. A small penetration may be sealed by proliferating epithelium, and a small localized
cataract may be the only result. However, a large perforation brings the
foreign proteins of the lens in sharp confrontation with the body's im-
munologic surveillance system, and opacification and severe inflammation ensues. The result, without surgical intervention, is usually a dense
cyclitic membrane, which may ultimately contract and tear off the ciliary
body. The outcome of such a sequence of events can be hypotony. In

the young eye, these reactions are faster and more aggressive. The attachment of vitreous body to lens capsule often draws the vitreous into the reaction, which ensures even greater inflammation. The statistics suggest that if vitreous is lost through a perforation, the result is somewhat akin to pulling a fire alarm. Perhaps it is the piezoelectric effect induced in hyaluronic acid when it is under tension (27). Armies of astrocytes, pigment epithelium, macrophages, and others charge out of the retina and hyalocytes are mobilized from the cortical vitreous, all for the purpose of forming tough fibrous bands across the interior of the eye. These cells will use retinal folds, vitreous collagen condensates, lens capsule, remnants of Cloquet's canal, the edges of a clot, and even ciliary processes for scaffolding. Once these bands form, anchor, and strength, they will contract and pull off the retina (9–17). The disorganized globe in the pathologist's bottle is the frequent end product of this apparently self-destructive process. Unhappily, we have not yet learned what chemical messengers and growth promoting factors start this series of events, nor what mechanism can be exploited to shut the process off. Thus, the strategy of the surgeon, as suggested in the book, *Intraocular Injuries* by Haik and Coles, is itself primitive and straightforward (17). The surgeon must anticipate the eye's natural subversion of the healing process and prevent it wherever possible. For example, the repair should be as atraumatic as possible so as not to aggravate the natural healing response.

Conditions that stimulate inflammation and fibrous should be excised. Thus, a ruptured lens should be totally removed. Vitreous in contact with any perforated area should be excised. Vitreous should be confined to the vitreous cavity. The vitrectomy procedure developed and perfected in the past 15 years has made this phase of repair possible (18–26).

All injured tissues should be repaired and returned to their normal locations so that abnormal adhesions do not get an opportunity to form. It is in these last categories that Healon has been of great help. It can coat and protect endothelium while lens fragments are removed from the eye. It will also prevent endothelial trauma while iris tears are repaired or cyclitic membranes are excised. As a dissecting instrument, a jet of Healon can gently tear away newly formed synechiae or dissect away clots. The presence of Healon can separate anterior chamber tissues and keep them in their proper anatomic positions. Thus, synechiae are prevented and final astigmatism may be minimized. Healon may also be used to replace excised vitreous and so fill the vitreous cavity with a more physiologic medium.

In the detailed description of corneal laceration repair to follow, the sections in which Healon is used are identified with an asterisk.

REPAIR OF CORNEAL LACERATION

Preliminary Considerations

Perform as many preliminary diagnostic tests as possible to see if a foreign body is present in the eye and orbit. For example, ophthalmic ultrasound might also identify the presence of intraocular hemorrhage as well as possible posterior perforation sites. Take specimens for culture and smear from the cul-de-sac and wound site and have the laboratory check for bacteria and fungi. Preoperatively, administer tetanus toxoid along with local and systemic broad spectrum antibiotics. Use intramuscular antiemetics to prevent vomiting. Whenever possible, general anesthesia should be employed for cases of ocular perforation. However, great care must be used in placing the endotracheal tube into the patient so that no coughing or gagging is produced. If lid edema or hemorrhage is present, a lid speculum will probably put unnecessary pressure on the globe. Such pressure may expel intraocular structures. Thus, we recommend considering the use of lid sutures. For lid suture placement make three continuous bites along the length of the upper lid (just beyond the lash margin) using a double armed 4-0 silk suture. Two vertical bites are then made deep in the lid tissue going from lid margin to lid fold and including tarsal plate. Specifically, one bite is made along the medial aspect of the lid with the needle in the medial end of the suture, and the other is made laterally with the other free needle. The same is now done on the lower lid. Traction is then applied on the nasal and lateral ends as well as the medial loop of the suture to open the eye.

*Iris Management

If iris has prolapsed into the laceration, there is a reasonable chance that damage to the muscles of the iris will take place and atonicity will result. Such an iris is apt to fall against the peripheral portion of the wound in the postoperative period unless a peripheral iridectomy is performed.

To perform a peripheral iridectomy, the limbal conjunctiva at the 1:30 or 10:30 position is grasped with a toothless forceps, and a small fornix-based flap is developed (a retracted fornix-based flap will allow better visualization of the structures in the anterior chamber than a limbus-based flap). The conjunctiva is dissected posteriorly for 3–4 mm. To perform a peritomy in a soft eye with a shallow to flat chamber, a rounded, sharp knife is used to slowly cut a groove at the limbus. Care should be taken to hold the scalpel handle nearly perpendicular to the sclera. Once a partial groove is made, the groove edge may be grasped with a fine, toothed forceps and the groove deepened until the anterior chamber is entered in a small area of the groove. To facilitate the deepening of the groove, the surgeon may place a fine suture the depth of the groove on either side of the initial incision. The assistant can now pull the wound apart, allowing the surgeon to slowly dissect into the anterior chamber against taut tissue. The final peritomy should be 3–4 mm long. Once the chamber is entered, the iris will appear at the incision. An attempt to prolapse it may be made by gently depressing the posterior lip of the wound. If iris is caught in the corneal laceration, prolapse may not occur. A fine, nontoothed forceps is used to grasp the iris and perform the peripheral iridectomy. A cannula is now placed on the Healon syringe and a gentle jet of Healon is run around the angle, pushing iris root posteriorly. This maneuver will lyse any newly formed peripheral anterior synechiae, as well as deepen the chamber. The deepening may also pull the incarcerated iris back into the chamber if the laceration site is first lubricated with Healon and the cornea (under the prolapsed iris) is gently depressed.

If the chamber deepening alone does not reposition the iris, the iris may be slowly stuffed back into the chamber with a spatula. Once most of the iris is replaced, the last bit of tissue is irrigated into the chamber with a few gentle jets of Healon. At this point, careful inspection is made of the laceration site and the iridectomy site. All iris tissue and any debris is cleared from both locations.

Next, the anterior lens capsule is inspected with high magnification. If there is a large opening in the capsule, a cataract will ultimately form. It would certainly be more prudent to perform an extracapsular lens extraction at this point than wait for the lens to swell and opacify in the postoperative period and be forced to operate a second time. If an extraction is necessary, it should be done through a limbal incision after the corneal laceration is repaired. However, if the lens capsule is intact or only a tiny puncture is seen, the lens should be left untouched.

Wound Closure

A sharp reverse cutting needle on a 9-0 or 10-0 nylon suture will close the laceration in the least traumatic fashion. The needle bite for each interrupted suture should be at $1/2$ to $1/3$ corneal depth and about 1–2 mm from the edge of the wound. The suture should be tied so as to just approximate the wound edges. Remember, the edges of the corneal wound will swell and make a well-approximated wound water tight. The peritomy over the iridectomy site should be closed with one or two 7-0 or 8-0 gut sutures and the flap pulled over the sutures and anchored in place with a cautery or catgut sutures (Figs. 1–6).

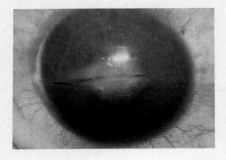

Figure 1. Preoperative appearance of eye (note iris prolapse through corneal laceration).

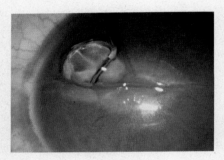

Figure 2. Placement of Healon into anterior chamber (top of eye at right).

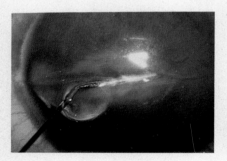

Figure 3. Further deepening of anterior chamber with Healon (top of eye at right).

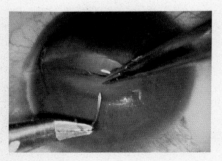

Figure 4. Placement of suture across the corneal laceration.

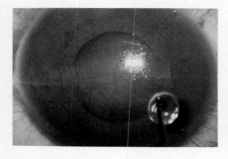

Figure 5. Final appearance of eye after completion of repair.

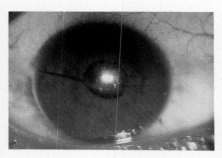

Figure 6. Follow-up appearance 3 months later.

Final Measures

At the close of the procedure, a subconjunctival injection of corticosteroids and antibiotics is given. The dressing should include an eye pad and firm plastic or metal shield. Postoperatively, local corticosteroids and antibiotics are given until successful healing is assured. Use of a short-acting mydriatic will help prevent the pupillary margin from sticking to the lens.

REFERENCES

1. Duke-Elder, S. *System of Ophthalmology Injuries. Part I.* vol. 14, p. 5, 6, 18-20, 421, 1972.
2. Eagling, E.M. Perforating injuries of the eye. *Br. J. Ophthalmol.* 60:732, 1974.
3. Snell, A.C., Jr. Perforating ocular injuries. *Am. J. Ophthalmol.* 28:263, 1945.
4. Moncreiff, W.F., Scheribel, K.J. Penetrating injuries of the eye: A statistical survey. *Am. J. Ophthalmol.* 28:1212, 1945.
5. Edmund, J. The prognosis of perforating eye injuries. *Acta Ophthalmol.* 46:1165, 1968.
6. Roper-Hall, M.J. Perforating ocular injuries: Prognosis. *Proc. R. Soc. Med.* 60:597, 1967.
7. Cinotti, A.A., Maltzman, B.A. Prognosis and treatment of perforating ocular injuries. *Ophthalmic Surg.* 6:54, 1975.

8. Adhikavy, H.P., Taylor, P., Fitzmaurice, D.J. Prognosis of perforating eye injury. *Br. J. Ophthalmol.* 60:737, 1976.

9. Schepens, C.L. Clinical aspects of pathologic changes in the vitreous body. *Am. J. Ophthalmol.* 38:8, 1954.

10. Constable, I.J., Tolentino, F.I. et al. Clinico-pathologic correlation of vitreous membrane, in Pruett, R.C., Regan, C.D.J. (eds): *Retina Congress.* New York, Appleton-Century-Crofts, 1974, p. 245.

11. Cleary, P.E., Ryan, S.J. Histology of wound, vitreous and retina in experimental posterior eye injury in the rhesus monkey. *Am. J. Ophthalmol.* 88:221, 1979.

12. Topping, T.M., Abrams, G.W., Machemer, R. Experimental double perforating injury of the posterior segment in rabbit eyes. The natural history of intraocular proliferation. *Arch. Ophthalmol.* 97:735, 1979.

13. Clarkson, J.G., Green, W.R., Massof, D. A histopathologic review of 168 cases of pre-retinal membrane. *Am. J. Ophthalmol.* 84:1, 1977.

14. Grabner, G., Boltz, G., Forster, O. Macrophage-like properties of human hyalocytes. *Invest. Ophthalmol. Vis. Sci.* 19:333, 1980.

15. Constable, I.J. Pathology of vitreous membranes and the effect of hemorrhage and new vessels on the vitreous. *Trans. Ophthalmol. Soc. U.K.* 95:382, 1975.

16. Kampik, A., Kenyon, K.R., Michels, R.G., et al. Epiretinal and vitreous membranes. *Arch. Ophthalmol.* 99:1445, 1981.

17. Haik, G.M., Coles, W.H. *Intraocular Injuries.* Philadelphia Lea & Febiger, Philadelphia, 1972.

18. Kasner, D. Vitrectomy: A new approach to the management of vitreous. *Highlights Ophth.* 11:304, 1968.

19. Machemer, R., Parel, J.M., Buettner, H. et al. A new concept for vitreous surgery: I. Instrumentation. *Am. J. Ophthalmol.* 73:1, 1972.

20. Machemer, R. A new concept for vitreous surgery: II. Surgical technique and complications. *Am. J. Ophthalmol.* 74:1022, 1972.

21. Kloti, R. Vitrektomie I. Ein neues Instrument für die hintere Vitrektomie, von Graefe. *Arch. Klin. Ophth.* 187:161, 1973.

22. Peyman, G.A., Dodich, N.A. Experimental vitrectomy: Instrumentation and surgical technique. *Arch. Ophthalmol.* 86:548, 1971.

23. Schepens, C.L. Vitreous surgery, in Pruett, R.C., Regan, D.J. (eds): *Retina Congress.* New York, Appleton-Century-Crofts. 1972, p. 677.

24. Aaberg, T.M., Machemer, R. Vitreous band surgery. *Arch. Ophthalmol.* 87:542, 1972.

25. O'Malley, C. Vitreous withdrawal as a therapeutic procedure. *Trans. Ophthalmol. Soc. U.K.* 71:773, 1951.

26. Ryan, S.J. Pars plana vitrectomy. *Trans. Am. Acad. Ophthalmol. and Otolaryngol.* 81:OP 352, 1976.

27. Barrett, T.W. Hyaluronic acid salt-A mechanoelectric transducer. *Biochim Biophy Acta* 385:157, 1975.

17
Blunt Trauma: Surgical Treatment of Hyphema Using Healon

Robert Stegmann

David Miller

Introduction

Generally speaking, rubbing the eye, even vigorously, does not produce damage to the internal structures. A vigorous rubbing indents the cornea and forces a responsive distention of the corneoscleral ring, giving the eye the shape of a vertical ellipsoid. When a firmly hit squash ball or a fast moving fist strikes the eye, the cornea is flattened or indented and the corneoscleral ring distends to give the eye the shape of a vertical ellipsoid. However, in this second case, marked internal damage can occur within the eye. The key difference between the two cases is the speed at which the distorting force is applied to the eye. With an eye rub, the force is applied slowly, and so the internal structures have a chance to readjust to the new position. An exploding champagne cork, however, applies a force that tears the internal structures before they have had the chance to shift or stretch. The combination of forces produced by rapidly stretching the eye into a new shape, along with driving the aqueous backward against the iris and lens, can effect every part of the eye. The eye tissue responds to the blow in three ways (1). First, the struck tissue seems to go into a state of shock and stops functioning for a while. More specifically, cells and fibers are stretched, cell membranes and organelles are disturbed, and function ceases. For example, a forceful blow by a fist bows the cornea backwards. The endothelial sheet

187

becomes stretched (2), junctions between cell clumps are pulled apart, and aqueous seeps into the corneal stroma, producing the typical central disciform edema seen after blunt injury. The second biologic response to a blunt, explosive force is vascular. The vasculature of the iris will dilate, perhaps in response to a rapidly secreted chemical mediator. Serum and cells will pour out of these distended, leaking vessels and produce the well-known cells and flare of traumatic iritis or Berlin's macular edema. Finally, the blunt force may be of such a magnitude as to actually lacerate tissue inside the eye. Thus, the root of the iris may tear and its severed blood vessels pour blood into the anterior chamber, the lens zonules may rip and the lens become subluxated, or lens opacities may form or some fibers of the iris sphincter may burst, producing a traumatic mydriasis. This latter constellation of changes are commonly grouped together in an entity known as the anterior traumatic syndrome of Frenkel (1). Of all the damage described in Frenkel's syndrome, the consequences of hyphema are the most serious. Not only can the immediate effect of blood in the anterior chamber drive the intraocular pressure to very high levels, but a future unrelating glaucoma can occur if the ciliary muscle is torn from its anchor at the scleral spur and a recession of the angle takes place. This latter problem will occur if the tear involves at least half of the angle circumference and is actually found in about 8% of patients sustaining traumatic hyphema (3). Of course, a severe hyphema in concert with elevated intraocular pressure can produce blood staining of the cornea. If this should occur, clearing of the cornea may not take place for months to years (4,5).

How should hyphema be managed? Most cases respond to five days of hospitalization, bed rest, and some form of symptomatic medical management. For example, one can use Diamox or timolol for increased intraocular pressure, corticosteroids and cycloplegia for the pain of iridocyclitis, and local antibiotics for an accompanying corneal abrasion. Is there a regimen that hastens the absorption of the blood? Havener (6) reviewed the subject in detail and concluded that "the spontaneous course of hyphema is totally unchanged by any form of medical management."

The major indications for the surgical removal of blood in the anterior chamber are as follows:

1. Uncontrolled glaucoma
2. Early blood staining of the cornea
3. Persistent total hyphema for more than nine days duration, which can produce anterior peripheral synechiae

It should be stressed that the surgical removal of clotted blood in the anterior chamber is a difficult and risky operation. Heroic removal of clotted blood can bring iris, ciliary body, or lens along with it.

If the clot has been present for a few days and is to be removed surgically, Healon can be very helpful. Jets of Healon used as a dissecting vehicle can gently break early peripheral synechiae.

In the detailed description of the removal of clotted blood from the anterior chamber, the sections in which Healon is used are identified by an asterisk.

SURGICAL REMOVAL OF CLOTTED BLOOD

Preliminary Considerations

The surgeon may use his or her usual method of preparation and draping of the patient as well as the most convenient mode of anesthesia. Either lid sutures or a favorite lid speculum may be used along with superior rectus stay suture placement.

Irrigation of the Anterior Chamber

A 180° conjunctival flap is developed superiorly. A fornix-based flap allows better visualization of the structures near the 12 o'clock position and may be taken down easily in the event that another hemorrhage develops. Entry into the anterior chamber is made along a 5-mm limbal incision. A rounded blade is used to gently scratch down into the anterior chamber. Since entry into the chamber is akin to entry into a dark room, movements should be small and done very carefully to avoid damage to vital structures. Once the chamber is entered, nonclotted blood will exit. A flat-tipped cannula on a saline-filled syringe is then placed on the edge of the scratch incision. The stream of irrigation is directed parallel to the iris plane covering the iris in all directions. Care must be taken to depress the lower lip of the wound in order to allow fluid to escape.

*Clot Removal

To get easy access to all the structures of the anterior chamber, the limbal incision is carefully extended for 180°. To deepen the chamber and keep vital structures away from the tips of the corneal scissors, Healon is slowly introduced before the incision is enlarged. The Healon will also coat the endothelium and protect it if instruments are introduced into the chamber to remove the clot or repair the iris. Once a large clot is identified, irrigation, forceps, and a vitrector are used to slowly dissect the clot from the tissue. Once most or all of the clots have been freed and rinsed away, the cannula on the Healon syringe is moved around the angle dissecting away all the newly formed synechiae in its path. Having restored the chamber structures to normal, a peripheral iridectomy is made at 12 o'clock.

Wound Closure

Since corticosteroids should be used if the postoperative period is stormy, wound healing will be slowed down. Thus, closure with nonabsorbable sutures is recommended. 9-0 or 10-0 nylon sutures applied in an interrupted fashion should be placed in a radial manner to close the incision. Before complete closure, Healon is irrigated from the chamber. The conjunctival flap can be tacked down at the wound edges with 7-0 catgut suture (Figs. 1–5).

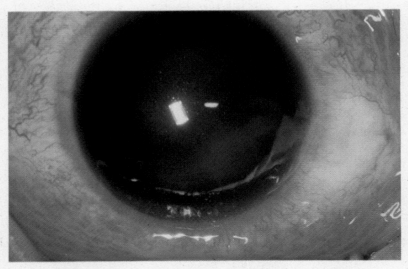

Figure 1. Preoperative appearance of the eye with hyphema.

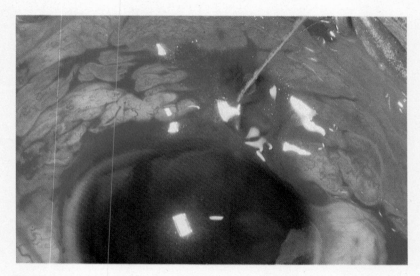

Figure 2. Introduction of Healon into anterior chamber through small limbal incision.

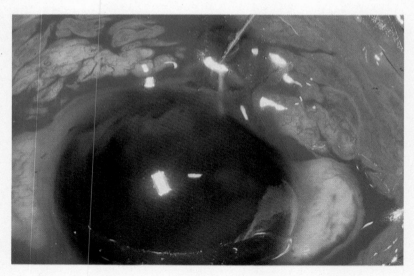

Figure 3. Lysis of angle adhesions using gentle jets of Healon.

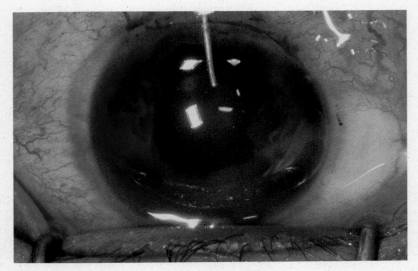

Figure 4. Appearance of anterior chamber filled with blood and Healon.

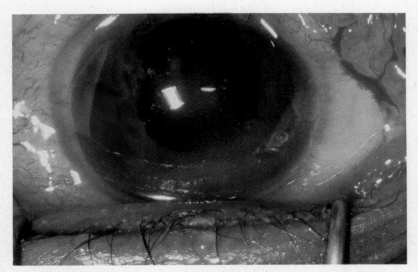

Figure 5. Appearance of the eye after as much blood as possible was safely removed and the limbal incision was closed.

Final Measures

At the close of the procedure, a subconjunctival injection of corticosteroids is given. Antibiotic ointment is then placed on the eye. The dressing should include an eye pad and firm plastic or metal shield. Postoperatively, local corticosteroids and antibiotics are given until successful healing is assured. Use of a short-acting mydriatic will prevent the pupillary margin from sticking to the lens.

REFERENCES

1. Duke-Elder, S. A System of Ophthalmology Injuries. St. Louis, C.V. Mosby.
2. Miller, D., Weiss, J.N. Endothelial Stretch. *Ophthalmic Surg.* 13:541, 1981.
3. Wilson, F.M., II Traumatic hyphema. *Ophthalmology* 87:910, 1980.
4. Brodrick, J.D. Corneal blood staining after hyphema. *Br. J. Ophthalmol.* 56:589, 1972.
5. Shammas, H.F., Matta, C.S. Outcome of traumatic hyphema. *Ann. Ophthalmol.* 7:701, 1975.
6. Havener, W.H. *Ocular Pharmacology*, 4th Ed. St. Louis, C.V. Mosby, 1978, pp. 330–341.

18

Sodium Hyaluronate (Healon) and Intraocular Pressure

Barry Kusman

Norman S. Jaffe

Henry M. Clayman

Mark S. Jaffe

Hyaluronic acid is an important component of the extracellular matrix of connective tissues such as vitreous, subcutaneous tissue, umbilical cord, synovial tissue, and synovial fluid (1).

In the human eye, sodium hyaluronate is a physiologic substance present in the aqueous humor and vitreous. Hyaluronic acid is tightly packed between the loose network of collagen fibrils, imparting rigidity and elasticity to the vitreous body. Its concentration is highest in the cortical layer where the hyalocytes responsible for its production are located (1).

Hyaluronic acid has been used successfully as a vitreous replacement after vitrectomy and retinal detachment surgery (1–6).

Healon has been developed as an ophthalmosurgical aid for various anterior segment procedures, such as intracapsular cataract extraction (ICCE), extracapsular cataract extraction (ECCE), intraocular lens (IOL) implantation, keratoplasty, and glaucoma surgery (7–10, 12).

Healon maintains a deep anterior chamber (AC) during surgery, allowing for more efficient manipulation and less corneal endothelial trauma during IOL implantation. It supports the iridovitreal or iridocapsular diaphragm and protects other surrounding tissues (7–10,16,18).

Healon for use in humans is obtained from rooster combs and is a highly purified 1% solution of sodium hyaluronate, which is supplied as a sterile, nonpyrogenic, nontoxic, transparent, viscoelastic preparation (1,6,7,9,10). It also appears to be noninflammatory, nonantigenic, and is thought to limit postoperative inflammation in the anterior chamber and to prevent formation of synechiae and adhesions (1,6–9).

Healon leaves the AC by way of the aqueous outflow channels (1). The viscosity of the substance has to be reduced by dilution with aqueous humor before this hydrophilic solution passes through the trabecular meshwork (16). Because Healon is about 98% water, it does not present a serious barrier to aqueous outflow. Other possible exit routes of Healon from the eye are via the vitreous, aided by the hyalocytes located in the cortical gel (1) and by resorption through the conjunctiva (specifically when used in filtering surgery).

One of the problems associated with the use of Healon is a transient rise in postoperative intraocular pressure (IOP). Certain factors need to be considered as possible contributions to this phenomenon:

A. Preoperative considerations
   1. Known family or personal history of primary or secondary glaucoma
   2. Anatomic anterior chamber angle anomalies
   3. Previous anterior segment inflammation or trauma (surgical or otherwise)
   4. Facility of outflow
   5. Prolonged use of medications influencing IOP, e.g., steroids
   6. Concurrent effect of preoperative medications, e.g., mydriatics, hyperosmotics

B. Surgical considerations
   1. Type of procedure performed, e.g., ICCE versus ECCE, glaucoma surgery, keratoplasty, vitreous replacement
   2. Site of incision
   3. Size of incision
   4. Enzymatic zonulysis
   5. Status of anterior hyaloid membrane
   6. Irrigation and/or aspiration of Healon

7. Presence of intraoperative complications, e.g., hemorrhage, vitreous loss, ruptured posterior capsule, inadequate aspiration of
   residual lenticular material
8. Incomplete or inadequate iridectomy

C. Postoperative considerations
1. Postoperative acetazolamide, timolol, or miotics
2. Postoperative hyaluronidase injection

Over the past few years several studies have been performed in humans to evaluate the effect of Healon on IOP.

Miller and Stegmann (9,10) used Healon to fill the AC after ICCE but
prior to the implantation of a Binkhorst iris clip lens in 20 eyes. They
found no significant increase in IOP in the Healon-treated eyes in the
first month postoperatively, as compared to the 20 fellow control eyes
in which air and saline were used in place of Healon.

Pape (12) studied 38 patients who underwent implantation of an iris
suture medallion-style lens, 35 after ICCE and three after ECCE. In the
ICCE group, 18 control cases had surgery performed under air or balanced salt solution (BSS), and in the remaining 17 cases 0.2 cc of Healon
was injected into the AC immediately upon entry into the eye. The AC
was fully reformed with Healon after the cataract extraction. In the first
10 ICCE Healon patients more Healon was injected to reform the AC
after IOL implantation, and it was not irrigated out. In the remaining
seven ICCE patients Healon was diluted by intracameral irrigation with
BSS before complete wound closure. All ICCE patients received intracameral acetylcholine (Miochol) at the end of surgery before wound
closure. In the three ECCE patients, Healon was also diluted before
complete wound closure.

In the ICCE Healon group, nine patients had IOP greater than 22
(ranging from 22–70 mm Hg) when Healon was not irrigated out. None
of the patients in this group had IOP greater than 21 mm Hg when
irrigation of the Healon was performed.

The sharp increase in IOP evident in the nonirrigated Healon cases
usually lasted from 24 to 48 hours, while dilution of intracameral Healon
appears to have abolished this postoperative elevation. At one to two
weeks and thereafter, the pressures returned to normal in all cases managed by either method. The pressure elevation resulting from Healon
is therefore thought to be only transient.

Several other studies have been performed using both ICCE and ECCE
techniques with the aid of Healon in IOL implantation (13–15,18,19).

All these studies confirm that failure to irrigate excess amounts of Healon out of the AC at the completion of surgery may result in moderate to severe transient elevations of IOP, which manifests in the first 24–48 hours postoperatively.

In another study by Stegmann and Miller (21), of 40 eyes undergoing ECCE by the Scheie technique (22), 20 eyes had the AC filled with Healon prior to the anterior capsulotomy and again during the irrigation and aspiration phase of the surgery. Twenty control eyes had the same procedure performed using Ringer's lactate as the irrigant. At the end of the procedure, remnant Healon (in the Healon-treated eyes) was left in the AC. No postoperative elevations of IOP were noted in either of the groups in this series, although the authors found that some patients undergoing the procedure have manifested a transient rise in IOP, probably related to the presence of Healon, that can be controlled with systemic acetazolamide or local timolol. Hence, they recommended that most of the Healon be replaced by BSS after suture closure.

Binkhorst (11) studied 20 patients in whom an ECCE with implantation of a 2-loop Binkhorst iridocapsular lens was performed. In 13 cases, 0.25 ml of Healon was injected into the AC after cataract extraction and before lens implantation. Healon was not irrigated out of the eye after surgery. Seven other control patients underwent the same procedure without the use of Healon. Intraocular pressure was recorded pre- and postoperatively daily for five days for the operated and fellow (unoperated) eyes in the Healon group and for the operated eyes in the control group. In the Healon group, 10 of the 13 eyes operated on had markedly elevated IOP during the first 24–72 hours postoperatively, despite the administration of acetazolamide and pilocarpine eye drops. However, the patients' fellow eyes displayed a slightly decreased IOP in the early postoperative period, possibly due to routine administration of acetazolamide. The control eyes also had slightly lower pressures postoperatively. Intraocular pressures fell spontaneously to normal in all cases except one, which required the administration of 0.5% timolol drops twice daily to normalize the pressure.

Another study (23) was performed on 107 patients who underwent cataract extraction and IOL implantation using phacoemulsification. Thirty-eight eyes had phacoemulsification performed in the AC followed by the insertion of a 2-loop Binkhorst iridocapsular lens under the protection of an air bubble. In a second group, 29 eyes had the same procedure performed using a Shearing single-plane posterior chamber lens. A third group of nine patients had a Shearing posterior chamber lens implanted under an air bubble, but the cataract removal was accomplished using phacoemulsification in the posterior chamber. In the last group of 31 patients, phacoemulsification was performed in the posterior chamber and a Shearing posterior chamber lens was inserted under an air bubble, but Healon was used many times throughout the procedure and was used to coat the surface of the IOL prior to insertion. Before wound closure, the Healon and air were irrigated out and the AC was filled with BSS. Pre- and postoperative IOP measurements were taken at two, seven, 15, and 30 days in all the Healon patients. Using this technique, there was no statistically significant difference between any of the mean pre- and postoperative pressures (Student's t test).

We have studied Healon and its effect on postoperative pressures using various modalities of ECCE surgery, with and without IOL implantation.

In all the groups studied initially, Healon was used to fill the AC prior to performing the anterior capsulotomy, as well as during nuclear prolapse and removal, either by expression or phacoemulsification. Healon still present in the chamber was then irrigated and aspirated out, together with the remnant cortical material, using automated equipment. When implants were inserted, Healon was used to coat the anterior surface of the pseudophakos and, when necessary, to fill the AC to facilitate pseudophakos insertion. At the termination of surgery, an attempt was made to irrigate and aspirate any remnant Healon out of the AC using BSS. As the studies progressed, we used lesser amounts of Healon during the different stages of surgery, to a point where Healon was only used in the later cases during pseudophakos implantation, and only when essential during earlier stages. In the control groups, BSS and air were used in all cases in place of Healon.

All our studies included pressure measurements by applanation tonometry at one and three days and six weeks postoperatively.

The first group consisted of 19 eyes undergoing standard ECCE. Seven eyes received Healon during surgery and 12 acted as controls. Average mean IOP for the Healon group was 29 on the first day, 17.1 on the third day, and 12.3 mm Hg at six weeks postoperatively. Corresponding values for the control group were 18.7, 13.0, and 14.4 mm Hg, respectively. The p values obtained revealed a significantly higher pressure in the Healon group on the first postoperative day ($p < 0.025$) as compared to values obtained on the third day and six weeks postoperatively, where p was < 0.1.

Phacoemulsification was performed on the second group of eyes in which six eyes received Healon and 12 eyes acted as controls. Average mean pressures in the Healon group were 21.8 on the first day, 13.3 on the third day, and 13.0 mm Hg six weeks postoperatively. Corresponding values in the controls were 16.2, 16.0, and 14.1 mm Hg, respectively.

Significantly higher p values were again obtained in favor of the Healon group only on the first postoperative day ($p < 0.01$).

Although the number of eyes studied in both groups is small, a definite trend is present, supporting higher postoperative pressures in the first 24–48 hours in those eyes receiving Healon.

Our third group, and the largest studied to date, consisted of 158 eyes undergoing planned ECCE with the implantation of a Shearing-type posterior chamber lens. Fifty-six of the eyes received Healon as outlined above, and 102 eyes acted as controls. Average mean pressure values in the Healon group were 23.3 on the first day, 16.9 on the third day, and 12.7 mm Hg at six weeks postoperatively, with corresponding values of 21.0, 16.5, and 13.7 mm Hg in the control group, respectively. The p values obtained in this group ($p < 0.05$) are in accordance with the results in our former two groups, as well as the experience of several other studies, and suggest that the ocular hypertensive effects of Healon are most pronounced in the first 24–48 hours postoperatively. By the third day and thereafter, this pressure elevation becomes statistically insignificant.

In our studies we noted that Healon did not result in obstruction of either the phacoemulsification or I/A tip of the automated equipment used.

Pape and Balazs (8) conducted a study using Healon in several types of anterior segment procedures, monitoring the IOP response in each.

ICCE was performed in 15 control patients and in 19 patients using Healon. In all 15 control cases, the AC was refilled with BSS after lens delivery. In the Healon group, 11 of the 19 patients received 0.3 ml of Healon after lens delivery and the remaining eight of the 19 patients received 0.2 ml of Healon on entering the AC; following the lens delivery the AC was reformed with approximately 0.3 ml of Healon. Postoperatively there was no specific rise in IOP in either group.

ECCE was performed in three control patients where BSS was used in the conventional manner, and in another three patients Healon was inserted to fill the AC immediately upon entry, and again at the end of the procedure. Postoperative IOP was the same in both groups of eyes.

Trabeculectomies were performed in 15 patients with medically uncontrollable glaucoma. Healon was injected into the AC at the end of surgery so as to fill the AC completely and extrude through the trabeculectomy site to extensively fill the subconjunctival filtration bleb. In two additional patients, a combined trabeculectomy/cataract extraction was performed using Healon in the same manner. In all cases the IOP was well controlled postoperatively without need for subsequent ocular hypotensive medications.

21. Stegmann, R., Miller, D. Extracapsular cataract extraction with Na-hyaluronate. Presented at the meeting of the American Intraocular Implant Society, Los Angeles, Calif., March 1981.

22. Scheie, H.G. Aspiration of congenital or soft cataracts: A new technique. *Am. J. Ophthalmol.* 50:1048, 1960.

23. Study KJH. Data on file at Pharmacia, April 1981.

19

Use of Healon in Vitrectomy and Difficult Retinal Detachments

Staffan Stenkula

Ragnar Törnquist

In posterior segment surgery the intravitreal approach has introduced a number of new problems. An unintentional damage of the retina, the optic nerve, or the posterior surface of the lens must be avoided, and certain demands concerning the technique are obligatory. These demands can be summarized as follows (1–4).

Maintenance of a Good Visibility of the Operative Field

The vitreous content should be substituted by a transparent product. Optical properties like those of the vitreous are also important, otherwise the inspection of the fundus may be hampered. If the operation is followed by a photocoagulation, these conditions are very important.

Maintenance of a Normal Intraocular Pressure

To keep the eye in a normal shape after vitreous removal, the intraocular pressure should be maintained at a normal level. If the pressure goes down, even a small vascular lesion can cause bleeding, which usually is stopped, however, by raising the intraocular pressure. The removal of the instrument from the eye involves risking a decrease of the intraocular pressure. This is particularly true if the substitute is a watery fluid.

Maintenance of the High Viscosity of the Vitreous Content

A leakage through the scleral opening is diminished or prevented if the vitreous substitute has a high viscosity. Also a high elasticity is advantageous so that the substitute can be injected through a thin cannula. A high surface tension is valuable for a blockade of a retinal hole. This quality may also prevent adhesion of surgical instruments to the substitute. A highly viscous fluid may have a damping effect on mobile intraocular structures (detached retina or retinal flap, intraocular foreign bodies, pieces of lens material in the posterior vitreous, etc.). In addition a viscous fluid can be used for separating a preretinal membrane from the retina or a retrolental membrane from the lens before removal. Blood is not easily mixed with a highly viscous solution, thus preventing an instantaneous spreading of a bleeding.

The above-mentioned conditions are fulfilled by Healon as a vitreous substitute because it has the following properties:

- Good transparency
- The same optical properties as vitreous
- High elasticity
- High viscosity
- High surface tension
- No toxic or allergenic side-effects

CLOSED VITRECTOMY

Introduction

In this operation microsurgical instruments are introduced into the vitreous cavity through the pars plana.

Instruments with a cutting and aspirating function (for instance, the Ocutome, Vitreous Stripper, VICS), scissors, hooks, and so on are used. One or two of these instruments are introduced into the eye at a time.

In the following situations Healon has proved to be of special value in closed vitrectomy.

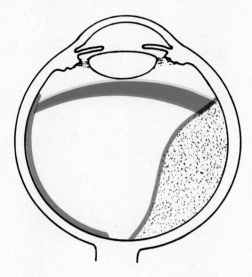

Figure 1. Retrolental membrane and a retinal detachment.

Excision of Retrolental Membranes

Retrolental membranes may develop after perforating injuries and intraocular inflammations. Removal of such a membrane during vitrectomy involves the risk of lens damage and a following cataract (Fig. 1).

Surgical Technique

The operation is initiated by preparation of a sclerotomy over the pars plana (4 mm from and parallel to the limbus using the Ocutome stiletto knive). A blunt 20-gauge cannula connected to a syringe with Healon is introduced into the eye between the retrolental membrane and the peripheral part of the lens under careful inspection through a contact lens and surgical microscope. When the tip of the cannula is in an ideal position, Healon is slowly injected so that the retrolental membrane is separated from the lens and easily removed with help of a vitreous cutter (Fig. 2).

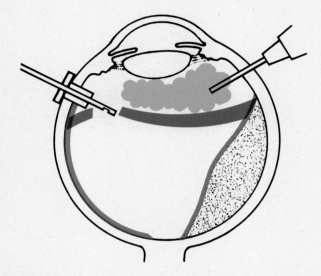

Figure 2. Healon injected between the lens and the vitreous membrane. A vitrectomy is performed.

Excision of Preretinal Membranes

Preretinal membranes are a common complication in many eye diseases (e.g., proliferative diabetic retinopathy, macular pucker, perforating injuries, and intraocular inflammation). Excisions of these membranes may lead to retinal damage and retinal detachment.

Surgical Technique

After excision of the vitreous in front of the retina, a 20-gauge cannula with a bent tip attached to a syringe with Healon is introduced into the eye through the pars plana 4 mm from and parallel to the limbus. The sclerotomy is prepared with the Ocutome stiletto knife. Under careful inspection the tip of the cannula is pushed under the preretinal membrane, and with the help of injections of small amounts of Healon, the membrane is separated from the retina and can be removed with a vitreous hook, cut with vitreous scissors or a vitreous cutter (Fig. 3). The procedure should be carefully done and, if necessary, repeated several times during the same operation.

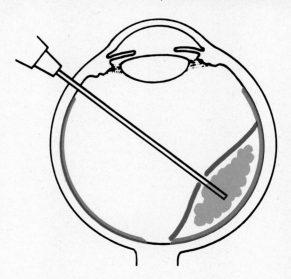

Figure 3. A preretinal membrane is elevated with a Healon injection and can safely be removed with a vitrectomy instrument.

Removal of Intraocular Foreign Bodies

Extraction of intraocular foreign bodies, especially fragments of non-magnetic material, involve great risk of retinal damage.

Surgical Technique

The vitreous is removed with the vitreous cutter so that the splint can be mobilized.

A blunt 20-gauge cannula attached to a syringe with Healon is pushed through a sclerotomy over the pars plana (prepared with the help of the Ocutome stiletto knife 4 mm from and parallel to the limbus), and a large "cushion" of Healon is placed around and over the splint. A sclerotomy large enough for passage of the foreign body is prepared. A microforceps is introduced through the scleral incision, and the fragment is mobilized and extracted. The "cushion" of Healon will prevent a possible bleeding from the retina to spread and disturb the visibility of the fragment. It will also protect the retina from further damage if the forceps should lose its grip and the fragment fall down to the bottom of the eye (Fig. 4).

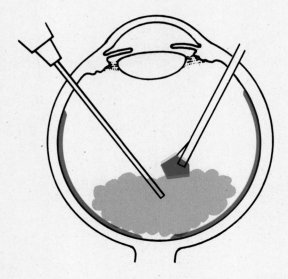

Figure 4. A "cushion" of Healon in the bottom of the eye during extraction of a foreign body.

OPEN SKY VITRECTOMY

Introduction

At present vitrectomy is generally performed according to the "closed" technique.

In cases with opaque cornea or very dense vitreous membranes the open sky technique is preferable. The operation involves complications in the form of retinal hemorrhage and choroidal detachment owing to the long-lasting low intraocular pressure. There is also the risk of collapse of the eye.

The use of a viscous vitreous substitute has been recommended in these cases (5).

Surgical Technique

A scleral supporter like Flieringa's ring is sutured to the sclera. A large button of cornea is removed with a corneal trephine. In phakic eyes the

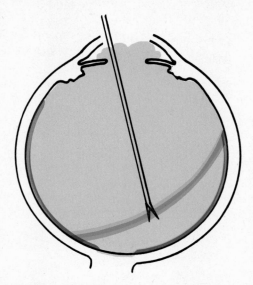

Figure 5. Open sky technique; cutting of a dense membrane.

lens is removed with a cryoextractor after an iridectomy. The microsurgical instruments can now be introduced into the vitreous cavity and opaque fibrous tissue can be removed. When material is aspirated from the vitreous cavity, an assistant injects Healon through a blunt cannula (Fig. 5). The observation of the posterior part of the eye is facilitated if a contact lens is used. A special contact lens that floats on the surface of the viscous material has been designed for this purpose (6). At the end of the operation the vitreous cavity and the anterior chamber is filled with Healon, and the corneal button is replaced or a corneal graft is prepared and carefully sutured using the general technique of corneal transplantation.

COMMENT

The use of watery fluids like saline and Ringer's solution as a vitreous substitute during vitrectomy has some disadvantages. Movements of elevated vascular membranes are not suppressed; this probably involves the risk of bleeding during and after the operation.

When a watery fluid is present in the vitreous cavity, even a small amount of blood spreads and may disturb the visibility of retinal details.

Thus, the viscous Healon may also prove to be of value as a vitreous substitute in "routine cases," as it gives support to mobile structures in the vitreous cavity and does not easily mix with blood.

RETINAL DETACHMENT

Introduction

In modern handling of retinal detachment there is a trend toward reducing the operation to an extraocular procedure where drainage of the subretinal fluid is avoided. The severe forms of retinal detachment with advanced vitreous changes or epiretinal membranes, however, need special surgical techniques, for example, intraocular surgery with excision of vitreous strands and membranes and reposition of highly detached retina and large retinal flaps.

In some of the surgical techniques the use of Healon has proved to be of great help.

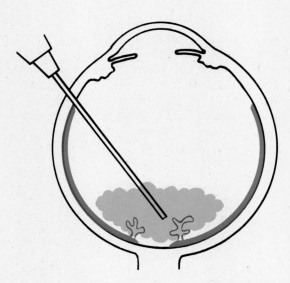

Figure 6. Immobilization of vascular membranes with the help of Healon.

High Bullous Retinal Detachment

In cases of very high bullous rhegmatogenous retinal detachment, it is difficult to place the scleral buckle in the correct position owing to the large amount of subretinal fluid. Adequate cryotherapy also gives problems in these cases as it is difficult to see the freezing effects through the subretinal fluid. Freezing time tends to become too long with risk of severe chorioidal damage.

Highly detached retina may flatten if the patient is immobilized for a few days. Unfortunately, this does not always happen, and immobilization often causes the patient great discomfort. Delaying the operation when the macula is detached may also lead to bad visual acuity.

The surgical procedure is facilitated if the highly detached retina is flattened out at the beginning of the operation. This can be achieved by drainage of the subretinal fluid. The eye generally becomes soft; thus, in order to perform the operation it is necessary to administer a vitreous substitute. If a fluent liquid like saline or Ringer's solution is introduced into the vitreous cavity, there is a risk of passage through the retinal tears. If, on the other hand, air is injected into the eye, there is less risk of passage through the retinal tears but visibility of the fundus is dis-

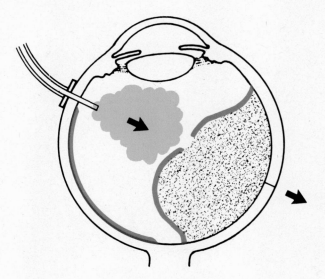

Figure 7. High bullous retinal detachment. Healon is injected into the vitreous cavity through the Ocutome cannula. Subretinal fluid is simultaneously drained.

turbed, especially if several gas bubbles are formed. The use of Healon highly facilitates the treatment of this type of retinal detachment (7).

Surgical Technique

The operation is initiated with a scleral incision using the Ocutome stiletto 4 mm from and parallel to the limbus. The infusion cannula (length: 2.5 mm) belonging to the Ocutome vitrectomy instrument is passed through the incision and fixed to the sclera with a preplaced 5-0 mercilene suture. By scleral impression and indirect ophtalmoscopy the tip of the cannula is checked to be free. The cannula is connected by silicone tubing to a syringe containing Healon. Thereafter the drainage of the subretinal fluid is performed using a thin 1.5 mm diathermy needle. When the subretinal fluid is released, Healon is slowly injected into the eye. Flattening of the retina is followed by indirect ophtalmoscopy. Two to four milliliters of Healon are generally injected before the retina is flat. Thereafter the operation is continued with treatment of the retinal tears. Whenever the intraocular pressure tends to be too low, small amounts of Healon may be injected into the eye. In order to avoid a too high intraocular pressure, the syringe with Healon can be removed between the injections. A careful aspiration of Healon may also be performed. By the end of the operation the cannula is removed and the sclerotomy is carefully closed using 7-0 Dexon (Fig. 7).

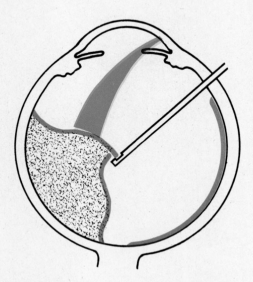

Figure 8. Accidental retinal damage during vitrectomy.

Mobile Detached Retina During Vitreous Surgery

When vitreous surgery is performed on an eye with mobile detached retina, there is a risk of accidental retinal damage when the retina is suddenly pulled against the cutting mechanism of the instrument (Fig. 8). The sudden movements of the retina can be hindered if the aspirated material from the vitreous is substituted with a viscous fluid such as Healon.

Surgical Technique

A sclerotomy is prepared 4 mm from and parallel to the limbus using the Ocutome stiletto knife. The Ocutome infusion cannula is inserted and fixed with a 5-0 Mercilene suture to the sclera. The cannula is connected to a syringe with Healon. The tip of the cannula is checked to be free by aid of scleral impression and indirect ophtalmoscopy. During excision and aspiration of the vitreous using a vitreous cutter, small amounts of Healon are injected into the eye through the cannula (Fig. 9). By the end of the operation the cannula is removed and the sclerotomy closed using 7-0 Dexon.

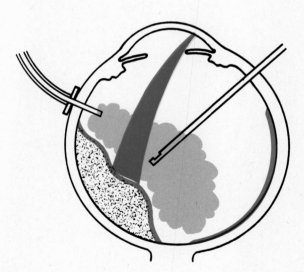

Figure 9. Immobilization of a detached retina during vitrectomy.

Giant Tears

The surgical treatment of retinal detachment following a giant tear with an inverted flap is complicated. Modern treatment of these cases includes a vitrectomy operation in which the vitreous is cut loose from the edge of the tear. Several techniques are described to push the flap of the tear back into its normal position, for example, gas injection. Healon may be of help for this purpose (8).

Surgical Technique

A closed vitrectomy is performed where all vitreous attached to the edge of the retinal flap is removed. A scleral incision 4 mm from and parallel to the limbus is made with aid of the Ocutome stiletto knife. A blunt 20-gauge cannula connected to a syringe of Healon is introduced through the incision, and a large cushion of Healon is placed on the bottom of the eye below the flap of the tear (Fig. 10). The watery liquid administered to the vitreous cavity during the vitrectomy (e.g., saline or Ringer's solution) is simultaneously released through the sclerotomy prepared

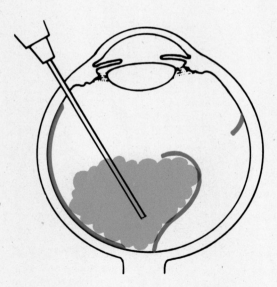

Figure 10. Giant tear with an inverted flap. A large "cushion" of Healon is injected under the flap.

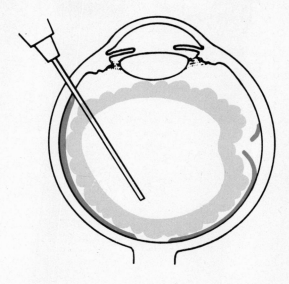

Figure 11. Large air bubble injected into the "cushion" of Healon in order to push the flap of the giant tear back against the wall of the eye.

for the closed vitrectomy using a fixed cannula (e.g., Vitreous stripper) or a mobile cannula (e.g., a "vacuum cleaner").

When the retinal flap has been pushed back into its original position, an additional injection of gas into the Healon cushion is performed. This will result in an air bubble stabilized by a layer of Healon that will keep the flap of the retinal tear in contact for several days and permit firm adhesions after cryo- or photocoagulation treatment (Fig.11).

COMMENT

Experimental studies (9) have shown that the viscosity of the vitreous has a great influence on the development of retinal detachment, since fluids with a low viscosity pass easily through retinal holes (Fig. 12). The administration of a viscous fluid in eyes with watery vitreous would reduce the risk of passage of fluid through retinal holes. Even resorption of subretinal fluid may be facilitated if the retinal holes are tamponaded by a viscous substance (Fig. 13). Therefore, Healon may prove to be of

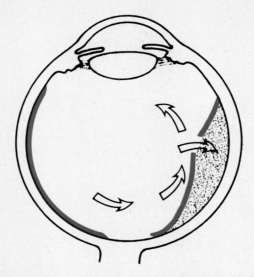

Figure 12. Movements in the vitreous with passage of fluid through a retinal tear.

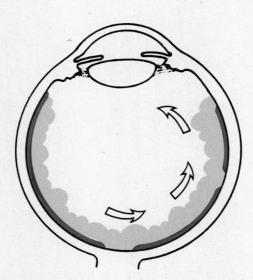

Figure 13. A layer of Healon slowing down the movements of fluid over the retina and tamponading the retinal tear.

value in the treatment of retinal holes, especially at the posterior pole where conventional technique is difficult.

REFERENCES

1. Balazs, E.A., Hultsch, E. in Irvine, A.R., O'Malley, C. (eds): *Advances in Vitreous Surgery.* Springfield, Ill., Charles C Thomas, 1976, pp. 601–602.

2. Klöti, R: Hyaluronsäure als Glaskörpersubstituent. *Ophthalmologica* 165:351, 1972.

3. Pruett, R.C., Schepens, C.L., Constable, I.J., Swann, D.A. Hyaluronic acid vitreous substitute, in Mac Kenzie Freeman, H., et al. (eds): *Vitreous Surgery and Advances in Fundus Diagnosis and Treatment.* New York, Appleton-Century-Crofts, 1977, pp. 433–434.

4. Eisner, R. *Eye Surgery.* New York, Springer-Verlag, 1980, pp. 174–178.

5. Pruett, R.C., Schepens, C.L., Swann, D.A. Hyaluronic acid vitreous substitute. *Arch. Ophthalmol.* 97:2325, 1979.

6. Schepens, C.L. Clinical and research aspects of subtotal open-sky vitrectomy. *Am. J. Ophthalmol.* 91:143, 1981.

7. Stenkula, S., Ivert, L., Gislason, I., et al. The use of sodium-hyaluronate (Healon®) in the treatment of retinal detachment. *Ophthalmic Surg.* (In press)

8. Kanski, J.J. Intravitreal hyaluronic acid injection. *Br. J. Ophthalmol.* 59:255, 1975.

9. Rosengren, B., and Österlin, S. Hydrodynamic events in the vitreous space accompanying eye movements. *Ophthalmologica* 173:513, 1976.

Index

Italicized page numbers refer to figures.

228   Index

transient, following lens implantation,
88
Globe, immobilization of, 32–3, 102, 123
Glycoprotein layers, 20, 21
Glycosaminoglycan secretion, 21
Guttata, corneal, 36

Healon (NIF-NaHA):
advantages of use, 23–24, 46, 48, 62,
67, 70, 92, 110, 120, 132, 142,
173, 181, 189, 195–196, 208
affected by red cell cytolysis, 19
amino acids in, 14
blood resorption and, 84
cellular infiltration and, 23
for coating instruments, 35, 36, 38, 62
for coating intraocular lens, 70, 74, *94*,
103, *105*
to deepen anterior chamber, *see*
Anterior chamber, deepening of
development of, 12–4
in dilation of pupil, 62, 64
distinguishing from vitreous, 40, *41*,
52–6, 111
in donor eye, *122*, 133, *134*
effect on cells, postoperative, 80
effect on implantation rated, 71
effect on visual acuity, 80, 82, 83, 100,
101
evaporation and, 48
exit routes from eye, 18–9, 96
formula of, 13–4
glycosaminoglycans in, 14
increase in intraocular pressure with,
196–202
inflammation and, 19, 23, 61, 84
injected into vitreous:
exit path, 18–9
residence time, 18–9
intravitreal hemorrhage and, 19
irrigation of, postoperatively, 40, 87,
197–8, 203
lysis of adhesions with, 112
macrophages and, 19
to maintain anterior chamber, *see*
Anterior chamber, maintenance
of
to maintain corneal shape, 43, 120, 126
manufacture of, 196
moisturizing effect:
on cornea, *42*, 48
on intraocular lens, 70, 74
molecular size, after injection into eye,
16
molecular weight, 14, 17
outflow after injection into eye, 88

to prolapse nucleus, 64
properties of, 208
to protect iris and lens, 33, 119
in reformation of anterior chamber, *see*
Anterior chamber, reformation
of
to replace aqueous humor, 14–16, *15*,
17, 62, 63
residence time, in vitreous, 18–19
to separate nucleus and endothelium,
64
surgical procedures using, 195
testing, 2, 13, 14
in trabecular meshwork, 88
use of compared with saline solution,
79–84
viscosity, 14, 17, 62
Hematoma, conjuctival, prevention of,
31–2, 48
Hemorrhage, 21, 99, 174, 182
intravitreal, 19
see also Bleeding
Hemostasis, 30
Heparin, 22
High-risk patients, 36
Hip joints, replacement, 109
Histiocytes, 20
Humans:
sodium hyaluronate in, 6, 14
trails of Healon in, 2
Hyalocytes, 7
Hyaloid:
bulging of, *86*
maintenance of, 114
Hyaluronic acid, *see* Sodium hyaluronate
Hydration, of epithelium, 20
Hyphema, 81, 188, *190*
management of, 188–9
Hypotony, 180

Incision:
closure of, *see* Wound, closure of
scratch, 144
small, advantages of, 59, 69. *See also*
specific tissues
Indomethacin, 70, 71
Inertness, biologic, 23
Inflammation:
caused by lens, 92, 111
caused by sodium hyaluronate, 5–6,
112
caused by trauma, 18
postoperative:
control of, 23, 84, 139
and lens adhesions, 109–110
side effect of Healon use, 19, 61, 84